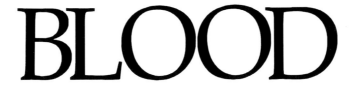

BLOOD

Atlas and Sourcebook of Hematology

SECOND EDITION

BLOOD

Atlas and Sourcebook of Hematology

SECOND EDITION

Carola T. Kapff, S.H. (A.S.C.P.)

Associate in Medicine, Harvard Medical School;
Supervisor, Hematology Laboratory,
Brigham and Women's Hospital, Boston

James H. Jandl, M.D.

George Richards Minot Professor of Medicine,
Harvard Medical School;
Physician, Beth Israel Hospital;
Senior Consultant in Medicine,
Brigham and Women's Hospital, Boston

Little, Brown and Company
Boston/Toronto/London

Library of Congress Catalog Card No. 91-62066

ISBN 0-316-48274-9

Printed in the United States of America

MV-NY

Dedicated to
Dr. William C. Moloney

Contents

Preface

In this age of dull automation, physicians, technologists, and other inhabitants of "heme labs" rely with pleasure on that most pragmatic of visual arts, blood morphology. The captivating colors and symbolic shapes of blood and marrow cells not only help relieve the gray tedium of poring over printouts but often provide keys to diagnosis and clues to pathogenesis.

This is primarily a color photographic atlas of blood and marrow as illuminated by the magical hues of Wright-Giemsa staining. In addition, appropriate attention is given special stains used in identifying cell lineage. Most lymphoma sections are rendered in H&E, whose deficient palette is enhanced by the useful artifacts of formalin fixation. A special section is devoted to the remarkable cells encountered in body fluids. Background coverage ranges from molecular biology to therapy, but no attempt is made to provide systematic pharmacologic information. Confusing or recondite terms are defined in the appended glossary.

We are indebted to Dr. David S. Weinberg, who provided most of the lymphoma sections, and to our mentor and friend, Dr. William C. Moloney, to whom this work is dedicated. The book would still be a stack of slides and foolscap were it not for the editorial skills of Nancy P. Jandl.

C.T.K.
J.H.J.

I. Examination of Stained Smears of Blood and Marrow

Assessing the Quality
of Wright-Giemsa Staining

Figure 1. Common Artifacts

Films of blood and marrow must be judged for quality of the smear and adequacy of staining. In evaluating a stained smear, one should first assess its general appearance and the suitability of staining; then, at low magnification, seek areas of the film that appear representative, display the entire polychrome spectrum, are free of artifact, and have the cells amply spread. **Figures 1-1** through **1-4** demonstrate common staining errors.

Viewed with the naked eye, a properly stained blood film is a pink smudge. Red cells should be pale reddish orange with a value close to blush pink. So-called "understained" red cells (**Figure 1-1**, ×800) actually appear excessively bright and colorful. That this smear is seriously understained is borne out by the faint pastel tints and vagueness of the leukocytes. The neutrophil nucleus should be a boldly defined purple, clearly distinguishable from the dappled lilac of the cytoplasm. Instead, this neutrophil nucleus is indistinct and blue and the cytoplasm rosy and featureless. The smear looks washed out. Understaining may signify any of several problems. A common one is excess acidity, often from acidic tap water, but other mischief may be at work: the buffer pH may have fallen below 6.4; the pH of the staining reagent may be incorrect; or acid fumes may have drifted into the work area. Often, understaining signifies shortening of the most vulnerable and capricious stage of polychrome staining—exposure of the smear to Wright-Giemsa after addition of water (or exposure to water-diluted Giemsa after the Wright stain). Although there are no eosinophils in **Figure 1-1**, eosinophil granules are excellent pH indicators, staining brilliant vermillion when the reagents are acidic and blue, taupe, or dark gray when they are alkaline.

The incongruous finding that red cells after staining have become green cells (**Figure 1-2**, ×800) commonly means that the smear is too thick. However, the cells in **Figure 1-2** are well and thinly distributed. An alternative possibility, that this overstained smear had been washed inadequately, is unlikely, for the background is clear. The most probable explanation is that either the duration of staining was excessive or the staining reagent or buffer was too alkaline (i.e., the pH was above 6.7). Unlike understaining, which makes the smear uninterpretable and necessitates restaining after the cause of the problem has been eliminated, overstaining does not necessarily preclude appraisal of the cells. Even khaki-colored red cells can be assessed for size and shape. The neutrophil at the top and the lymphocyte near the bottom appear unduly dark, but their identities and individual morphologic features remain readily ascertainable despite the artifact of alkalinity.

An example of a blood smear blotched by heavy deposits of oxidized stain is shown in **Figure 1-3** (×2,000), which reveals heavy granular precipitates of metachromatic dyestuff both on and between the cells. This problem can be obviated by passing the staining reagent through a filter before use, although it is better practice to use fresh reagent free of precipitate. When staining reagents leave sparse, fine deposits on the blood smear, these may very easily be mistaken for inclusion bodies, or the red cells may appear to be parasitized or infected. That such misinterpretations are quite possible is illustrated here by the tendency of the precipitates to adhere to the surfaces of cells, creating an illusion that many particles are intracellular or are bulging from the cell membranes. Occasionally, dye precipitated onto red cells may exactly sim-

ulate supravitally stained red cells containing Heinz bodies. A common error that will eventuate in deposition of precipitated dye, even though the reagent itself is fully solubilized at the time of its addition, is use of an inadequate volume of undiluted stain. If fewer than approximately 15 drops of stain are added to a standard (22 mm square) coverslip, or if the coverslip is not completely covered with liquid, a portion of the stain may dry ineluctably onto the glass. Whether coverslips or slides are used, one should take all reasonable precautions to assure that there is no appreciable evaporation of the dye solvents. After the second stage of the staining procedure, it is important to rid the coverslip or slide of diluted stain by flooding with water or by immersion but not by decanting.

Presence of water in the methanolic solution of Wright stain or condensation of moisture on the surfaces of blood smears before their fixation introduces distinctive artifacts (**Figure 1-4**, ×2,000). When telltale water bubbles are found in red cells throughout the smear, no attempt should be made to interpret the morphology, for water introduces treacherous artifacts capable of deceiving the sharpest observer. Were it not for the presence of refractile water bubbles, the red cells would be misconstrued as being small, hypochromic, and crenated: these are all shrinkage artifacts and simulate changes found in excessively thick blood smears. Moisture collects on red cell contours like beads of sweat. Lymphocytes are puckered by moisture. As illustrated by the lymphocyte in **Figure 1-4**, the cell is shriveled, and its cytoplasm—scant as it may have been originally—is now represented merely by a few wisps and flaps. The normal-looking band neutrophil attests that moisture has little or no effect on that juicier cell type. Moisture or water vapor may, however, decolorize the granules of unfixed eosinophils and basophils.

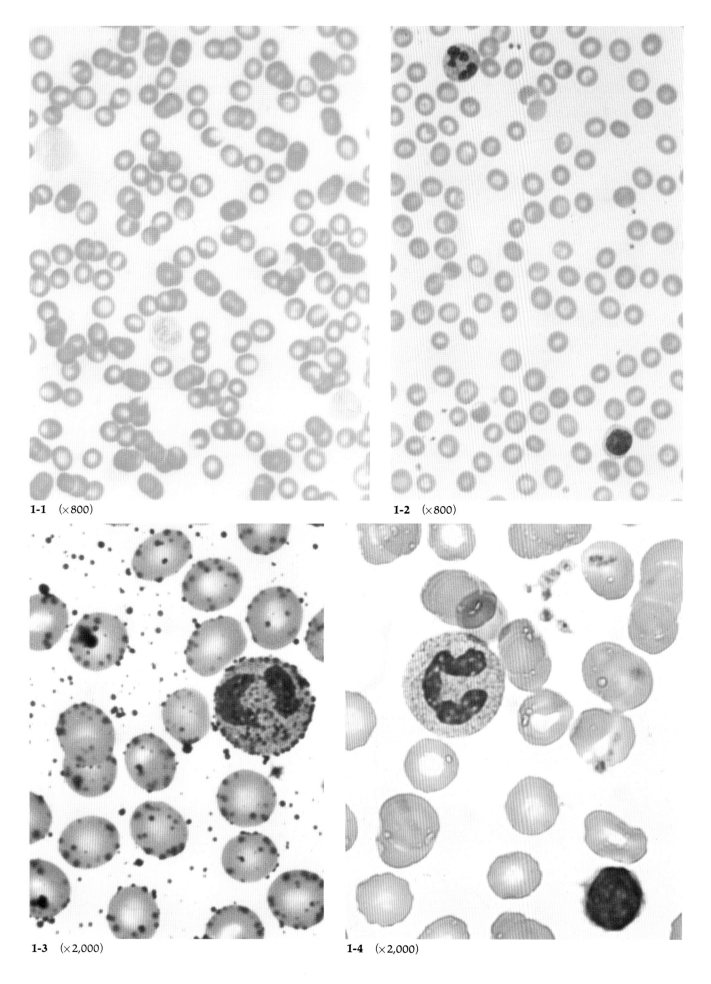

1-1　(×800)

1-2　(×800)

1-3　(×2,000)

1-4　(×2,000)

Selection of Good Areas for Inspection

Figure 2. Suitable Dispersion of Blood and Marrow Cells

More information can be obtained by examining the blood smear than by any other single medical procedure. Competence in examining smears of blood and marrow clearly is strengthened by supervised trial-and-error learning, but no special faculties are needed beyond sharpness of vision. One must develop a knack for selecting promising areas for concentrated inspection and for avoiding the "bad" areas present in virtually all blood smears. Each smear should be examined first with a 10× objective lens to seek out fields where cells are evenly spread. By inspecting a "good" area, the viewer may estimate the proportion of red cells, leukocytes, and platelets and thus be prepared to recognize any important departure from the expected in other laboratory reports. With experience and adoption of a systematic scanning ritual, the observer can assess red cell and platelet morphology, as well as the more conspicuous aspects of leukocytes, during this low-power survey. It is good practice to ascertain initially the quality of the smear and to confirm with a 40× objective that most red cells have a normal, biconcave shape, before switching to the oil-immersion lens. An uncrowded, well-spread, and well-stained smear is shown in **Figure 2-1** (×800). The red cells are light orange-pink and display normal areas of central pallor spanning half the cell diameter. In this field, the cells show slight variation in size but no undue variation in shape. The neutrophil is among the minority having four (rather than the customary three) segments, but it is undisrupted, free of vacuoles, and normal in size. The color of the nucleus and cytoplasm is representative. Evaluation of cytoplasmic granularity requires inspection with an oil-immersion lens. The half-dozen, well-dispersed platelets seem normal. At center right, a platelet overlies a red cell. As platelets have a colorless, but structural, halo (clear zone) about them, their appearance when perched upon a red cell may mimic an inclusion body or an intracellular parasite. A platelet impressed on a red cell often displaces enough hemoglobin to obliterate the central pale area, as shown here.

At the periphery of smears made on coverslips or slides, there is a size-determined maldistribution of cell types, with an unrepresentative overabundance of the largest blood cells. Red cells deposited at the outer edge of the smear are deformed into shapes that can mislead viewers not adequately suspicious of peripheral areas. Red cells at smear margins display 3 conspicuous features: they appear flattened, cornered, and lacking in central pallor (**Figure 2-2**, ×800). Wherever they abut they tend to have polygonal or faceted profiles. Flattened cells sometimes simulate spherocytes, but their largeness and normal color contradict this illusion. Crowding of several red cells into the band neutrophil at the bottom of the figure is characteristic of marginal artifacts as well as of smears that have partially dried before coverslip separation. If the entire smear resembles the scene depicted in **Figure 2-2**, the smear and its partner should be discarded and replaced by a different pair prepared from the same sample.

Figure 2-3 (×800) illustrates one of the common problems preventing evaluation of cell morphology. This smear was spread from an excessively large droplet of blood and is too thick with cells. In thick smears the red cells become superimposed, form extensive rouleaux, and shrivel during the protracted drying period. Thickly smeared cells may stain gray-brown, green, or blue. Furthermore, when red cells are amassed, aberrations in size and shape are concealed. The leukocytes and platelets also appear dark, primarily because of shrinkage during prolonged drying. The extent of deformation from shrinkage is attested to by the puckered neutrophil at the midright. Only with imagination can the wizened cell at top be identified as a monocyte.

The colorful, but uncrammed, appearance of a properly spread normal marrow aspirate is shown in **Figure 2-4** (×200). Competence in reading marrow films requires alertness to the tricky artifactual simulations of which excessively thick marrow smears are capable. With marrow, it is even more important than with blood to devote ample time to a preliminary search at low magnification and to examine each of the paired smears prepared from each specimen. The good quality of most of this low-power view invites more careful scrutiny at a higher power. Where cellular elements are jammed together, however, as in the dark stromal regions at the lower left, close examination would be fruitless. The marrow aspirate shown in **Figure 2-5** (×200) was spread thickly to compensate for the paucity of cellular marrow. This introduced thick-smear artifacts that hinder identification of most cells. Despite the soupy morphology, it is possible to assess overall cellularity crudely by noting the relative space occupied by fat cells (lipocytes). Allowing for skip areas characteristic of smeared aspirates, one can judge cellularity to be about half that in **Figure 2-4**. For an accurate appraisal of cellularity, the intact geography of biopsy material must be examined. At first glance, the shortcomings of the marrow smear depicted in **Figure 2-6** (×200) are inapparent. On closer inspection, it is clear that red cells are wadded together and heaped on the shriveled marrow cells. Finding thick piles of red cells should nudge one to move on to better-spread areas.

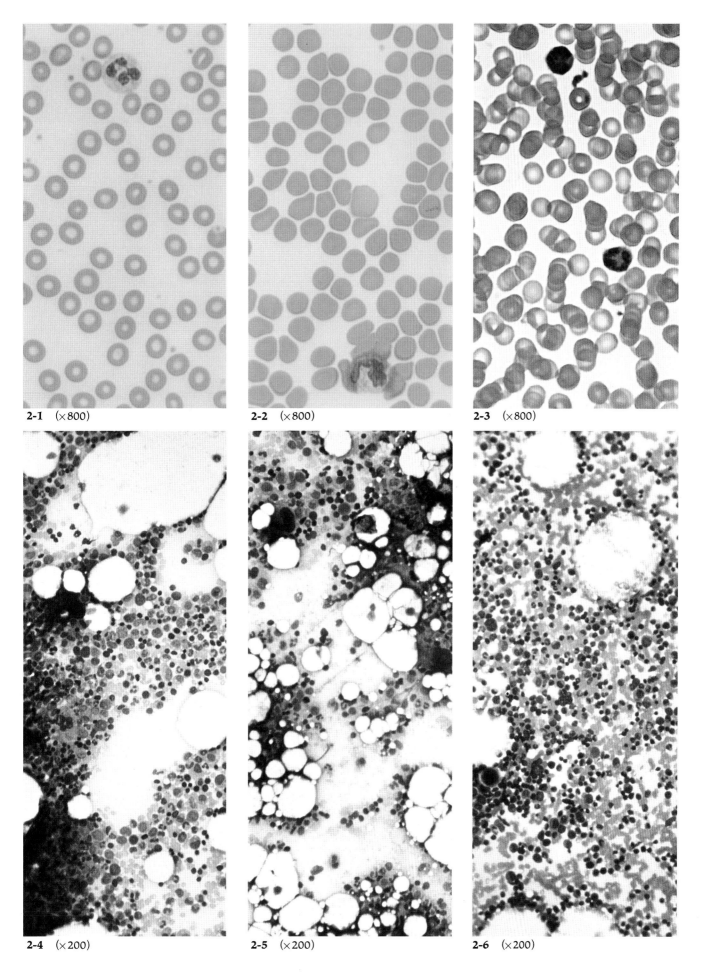

2-1 (×800)

2-2 (×800)

2-3 (×800)

2-4 (×200)

2-5 (×200)

2-6 (×200)

Normal Marrow

Figure 3. Myeloid Cells

The nomenclature applied to the hierarchy of precursive marrow cells is befuddled by redundant use of the term *stem* to define progenitor cells regardless of rank and level of stemhood. Stem cells, by definition, have two capabilities: (1) replication and (2) generation of more differentiated "daughter" cells. The ancestor of all blood cells is the multipotential hematopoietic stem cell, which begets two subordinate lines of pluripotential daughter cells. One generates all lymphoid cells: T cells, B cells, and natural killer (NK) cells. The other pluripotential stem cell is parent to 4 low-echelon committed stem cell lines, restricted in their potential to form only myeloblasts, monoblasts, proerythroblasts, or megakaryoblasts. **Figure 3** displays the myeloblast and its progeny.

A characteristic young *myeloblast* is depicted at the center of **Figure 3-1** ($\times$2,000). For comparison, examine the classic proerythroblast at the center of **Figure 3-2** ($\times$2,000) and the older myeloblast just above another proerythroblast in **Figure 3-3** ($\times$2,000). Myeloblasts have large, slightly oblong nuclei, eccentrically surrounded by narrow rims of blue cytoplasm but often containing small numbers of red granules. The nuclear chromatin is lavender pink, finely granular or softly stippled, sometimes sievelike, with 2 to 5 pale, often punched-out or perforate nucleoli. The nuclear membrane is finer than in lymphoblasts. Clumping of perinucleolar chromatin becomes evident in young *promyelocytes* as they acquire bold reddish (primary, azurophilic, or nonspecific) granules, which often overlie the nucleus (**Figure 3-4**, $\times$2,000). *Primary granules,* when abundant, certify maturation to the promyelocyte stage.

All maturational stages of promyelocytes are displayed in **Figures 3-4** through **3-6** (all $\times$2,000). As is seen in **Figures 3-4** and **3-5**, primary granules are prone to overlie the nucleus and, when numerous, may obscure it. With maturation, primary granules number in the dozens, and the cell enlarges to a diameter of about 20 μm, becoming larger than its parent cell, the myeloblast. At this stage (**Figure 3-6**, upper left), the copious cytoplasm normally retains a bright blue color, and the nucleoli are encroached on by the prominent cytoplasmic granules. The nucleus is displaced off center as the cell develops a fat cytoplasmic belly in the Golgi region. Promyelocytes undergo division, as do their offspring, the myelocytes, but synthesis of new primary granules ceases. The number of primary granules per cell is halved several times, and by the late myelocyte stage the number of primary granules per cell is comparatively small. The maturational changes during progression from promyelocyte to mature myelocyte are exemplified by the 4 large cells displayed (proceeding from top left to bottom right) in **Figure 3-6**.

By definition, the appearance in the cytoplasm of the variously colored *specific granules* (neutrophilic, eosinophilic, or basophilic) marks the cell as a *myelocyte*. The profusion of granules of both kinds combined may be sufficient to conceal the cell nucleus, the nucleoli (if any), and much of the cytoplasm. On completing their maturation-division steps, the maturing myelocytes (the large cell at the upper left in **Figure 3-1** and the two cells on the right in **Figure 3-5**) contain comparatively few granules, cytoplasmic basophilia is lost, and nuclear chromatin is coarsened. **Figure 3-4** (upper right) portrays a late myelocyte having some of the features of its more mature derivative, the *metamyelocyte*: the cytoplasm reveals a soft pinkish blush, the nuclear chromatin is distinctly condensed, and the eccentric nucleus is oblong and slightly flattened on its Golgi aspect. At the lower right of this figure and the upper left of **Figure 3-2** are several metamyelocytes, each of which shows a gentle medial indentation of the reniform nucleus. Metamyelocytes are smaller than myelocytes and much smaller than promyelocytes, the diameter (14 to 16 μm) only slightly exceeding that of band forms and segmented neutrophils. Metamyelocytes are the youngest nondividing cells of the granulocyte lineage. The chromatin of their bean-shaped nuclei is coarsely condensed, and the subdued cytoplasmic pinkness is comparable to that of mature granulocytes.

The derivative of the metamyelocyte is the *band form*. In this stage, the cell has achieved its final dimension (diameter, 13 μm): the nucleus is elongated, may have the shape of a sausage or horseshoe, and has a nearly constant transverse diameter of 3 to 4 μm. The chromatin is aggregated into evenly dispersed clumps about 1.0 to 1.5 μm across. The 2 band forms at the midleft in **Figure 3-6** possess both primary (large, dark purple) granules and specific (smaller, lilac-colored) neutrophilic granules in roughly a $1:8$ ratio. For comparison, note in this figure the young metamyelocyte and, at right center, the mature three-segmented *neutrophil*.

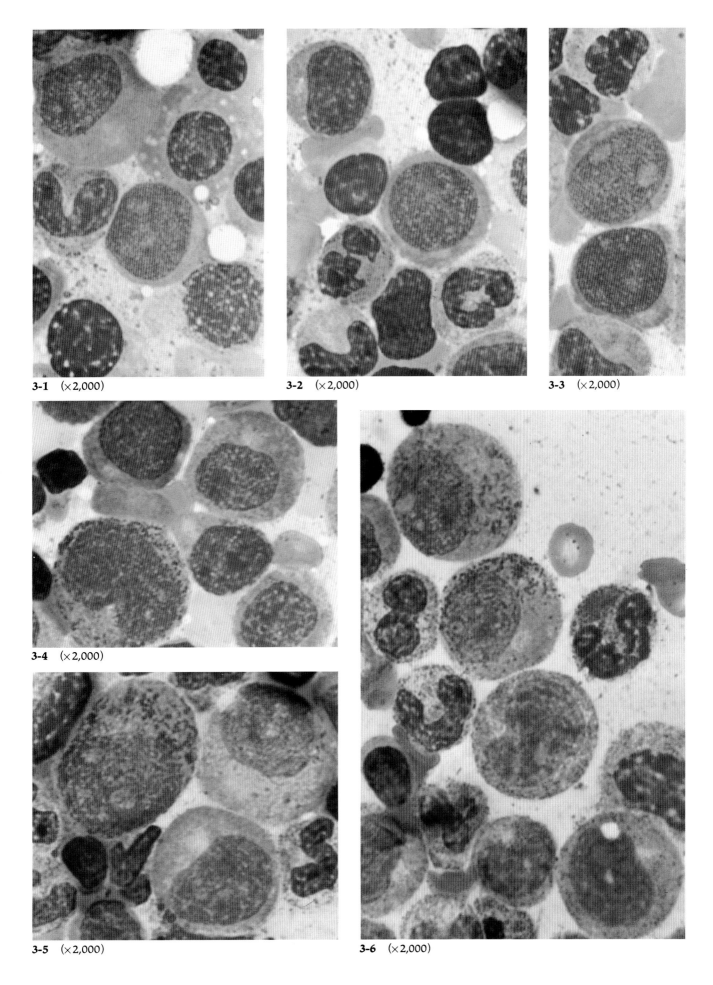

3-1 (×2,000)

3-2 (×2,000)

3-3 (×2,000)

3-4 (×2,000)

3-5 (×2,000)

3-6 (×2,000)

Figure 4. Erythroid Cells

The remarkable constancy of red cell levels depends on hormonal regulation of unipotential stem cell precursors of the earliest erythropoietic cells, the proerythroblasts. Erythropoiesis is governed by the hormone *erythropoietin*, which is released by renal vascular endothelium in response to hypoxia. Erythropoietin binds to receptors on erythroid colony forming units in marrow (CFU-Es) and instructs them to generate proerythroblasts. Generation by proerythroblasts of eightfold their number of mature, anucleate red cells is the end result of 3 successive division steps, followed by inactivation and ejection of the nucleus and, lastly, by the completion of cytoplasmic maturation. This series of transformations involves 5 morphologically distinct transitional stages. The cell types (and their aliases) representing these sequential stages are as follows: *proerythroblasts* (pronormoblasts); *basophilic erythroblasts* (basophilic normoblasts); *polychromatophilic erythroblasts* (polychromatophilic normoblasts); *orthochromatic erythroblasts* (orthochromatic normoblasts); and *reticulocytes*.

At the center of **Figure 4-1** ($\times 2,000$) is a normal young proerythroblast, the first cell of the erythropoietic series to synthesize hemoglobin. Normally, proerythroblasts constitute 2 to 3% of the erythropoietic cell population. Proerythroblasts, the largest of erythropoietic cells, achieve their maximum size (diameter, about 18 μm) as they prepare to enter prophase (**Figure 4-3**, $\times 2,000$). Initially, the proerythroblast is slightly oblong and has a large, nearly round nucleus occupying approximately 70% of the cell area. Unless displaced by neighboring cells, the nucleus is centrally situated, surrounded by deep blue cytoplasm devoid of granules. In the earliest proerythroblasts, the cytoplasm is clear unblemished blue, except for a thin discontinuous perinuclear clear zone. During maturation, the cytoplasm of cells at this stage becomes more darkly basophilic; an eccentric, often flaring, perinuclear corona appears; and in some regions, the deep blue cytoplasmic color becomes lightly mottled with yellowish pink. Even in the least mature proerythroblast, the nuclear chromatin is granular or branny and its reddish purple color is darker than the glassy, pale lilac chromatin of myeloblasts. Most proerythroblasts lack an obvious nucleolus. Sometimes there may be 1, or at most 2, indistinct bluish nucleoli having vague margins that fail to give the craterlike or punched-out appearance seen in other blast forms.

The daughter cell of the proerythroblast is the basophilic erythroblast (**Figure 4-2**, $\times 2,000$). Basophilic erythroblasts, which constitute 6 to 8% of erythropoietic cells, are round or slightly oblong and distinctly smaller than proerythroblasts (diameter, 12 to 14 μm). Most of the cytoplasm is medium blue, although the outer margin may be deeply basophilic. A pale, faun-colored perinuclear halo may be prominent. As in most erythropoietic cells, the nucleus is round and the nuclear membrane is sharply demarcated. The contained chromatin is more darkly purple and more coarsely clumped than in proerythroblasts. At the lower right of **Figure 4-4** ($\times 2,000$) is another basophilic erythroblast with similar dimensions but displaying as yet no perinuclear clear zone. Its identity is affirmed mainly by the coarsely aggregated purple chromatin of its nucleus. The cell type most easily confused with the basophilic erythroblast is the plasma cell, an example of which is conveniently adjacent (to the left of the erythroblast). The features that set plasma cells apart are as follows: their nuclei are small and often so eccentrically placed as to appear to be leaving the cell; the chromatin is grossly clumped; and the cytoplasm is copious, of a peculiarly opaque blue-gray color, and contains secretory vacuoles or inclusions.

The polychromatophilic erythroblast, descended from the basophilic erythroblast (and granddaughter of the proerythroblast), possesses a smaller, more condensed nucleus than its parent, with nuclear chromatin arranged in evenly spaced chunky aggregates that form clocklike patterns. The coarsely condensed chromatin imparts to the nucleus a blue-purple hue that is unique to erythropoietic cells. As demonstrated by the polychromatophilic erythroblasts in **Figures 4-2** and **4-5** ($\times 2,000$), the regularity and chunkiness of the nuclear chromatin clearly differentiates them from basophilic erythroblasts and proerythroblasts. The polychromatophilic erythroblast directly below the basophilic erythroblast in **Figure 4-2** demonstrates the cartwheel pattern that, on Wright-Giemsa stained smears, is more characteristic of these cells than of plasma cells. The outstanding cosmetic feature of the abundant cytoplasm is its muddy blue color. Except for the light pink perinuclear halo, most of the cytoplasm has an opaque, bluish tan hue. This represents the admixture of two complementary colors—the blue of stained RNA and the yellow-red of eosin-stained hemoglobin—which gave rise to the term *polychromatophilic*.

Orthochromatic erythroblasts (alias *normoblasts*) are the nondividing offspring of polychromatophilic erythroblasts. Orthochromatic erythroblasts represent two-thirds of marrow erythropoietic cells. Together with the polychromatophilic erythroblasts, these constitute 90% of the total erythropoietic population. Because of their pyknotic purple-black nuclei and abundant eosinophilic cytoplasm, the 4 orthochromatic erythroblasts in **Figure 4-5** are readily identifiable. After orthochromatic erythroblasts have expelled their inactivated pyknotic nuclei—often following nuclear fragmentation *(karyorrhexis)*—most newly anucleate red cells still retain (for a few more hours or days) some bluish coloration, for which they are termed *polychromatophils*. Note in **Figure 4-6** ($\times 2,000$) that about one-third of the cells are slightly larger than the others and lack central pallor. Most of these display the dusky, faintly gray-blue tinge typical of polychromatophils. As discussed under **Figure 17**, the ribosomes of most polychromatophils undergo aggregation during supravital staining with new methylene blue, permitting their enumeration as *reticulocytes*.

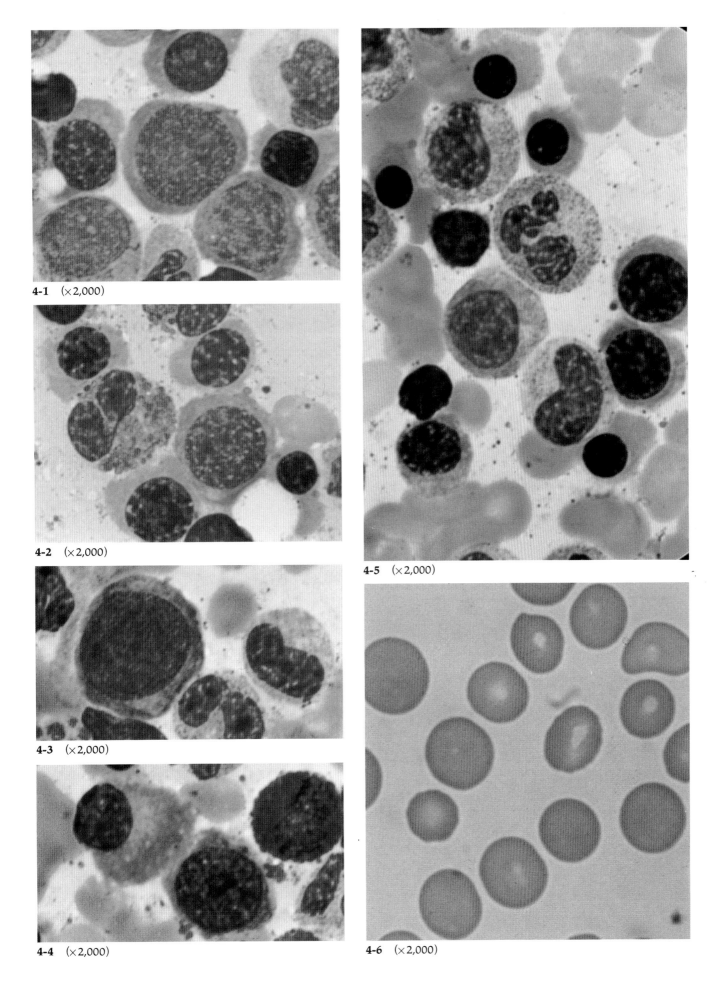

4-1 (×2,000)

4-2 (×2,000)

4-3 (×2,000)

4-4 (×2,000)

4-5 (×2,000)

4-6 (×2,000)

Figure 5. Megakaryocytes. Eosinophil Myelocytes. Plasma Cells.

The largest marrow cells are *megakaryocytes* (**Figures 5-1,** ×1,260 and **5-2,** ×800); these generate all blood platelets but represent fewer than 0.1% of all marrow cells. Mature megakaryocytes are multilobular—not multinucleated, as are osteoclasts of bone, Langhans giant cells of tuberculosis, or Reed-Sternberg cells of Hodgkin's disease—and each lobule possesses a diploid set of chromosomes. The precursive *megakaryoblasts* are 20 to 30 μm across and have large, rounded, dark purple nuclei surrounded by a rim of basophilic cytoplasm. As young megakaryoblasts mature, nuclear chromatin darkens and the nucleus undergoes endoreduplication (endomitosis). The number of lobules doubles during each of 3 endoreduplication steps, culminating in a huge polyploid cell possessing 8 lobes connected in series and measuring 60 to 100 μm across. Some megakaryoblasts undergo a fourth endoreduplication, yielding a cell with 16 connected lobes and 32 or even 64 sets of chromosomes. Further lobulation without synthesis of additional DNA occasionally occurs. This is hypersegmentation, not excessive endoreduplication, and is usually indicative of a megaloblastic process.

At the top of **Figure 5-1** is a *promegakaryocyte* caught in the act of endoreduplication. The 2 outer lobes are vertically segmented. The larger middle nuclear mass appears to be cleaving laterally into 2 lobes, bringing the total to 4. Normally, megakaryoblasts have several nucleoli, but none is visible here. Note the blueness of the exposed cytoplasm, its grainy texture, and the fringe of blue pseudopods, which are often visible in developing megakaryocytes. Proliferating populations of young mononuclear megakaryoblasts (as may be encountered in acute megakaryoblastic leukemia) can resemble large myeloblasts or lymphoblasts, but the presence of their pseudopodal "ears" is often a clue to identity.

The marrow from a patient with thrombocytopenic purpura in **Figure 5-2** is crammed with megakaryocytes. This crowded scene displays 8 of these physiologic giant cells, 2 of which are comparatively small megakaryoblasts. At center is a bilobed promegakaryocyte in which the wormy appearance of the nuclear chromatin, conspicuous nuclear membrane, and dark purple hue of the chromatin are all quite visible. This young cell also displays the first blush of cytoplasmic eosinophilia and a beginning granularity in the central hof that heralds the start of intracytoplasmic partitioning into platelet territories, preparatory to release of intact platelets. Above and below this cell are 2 nearly mature, 8-lobed megakaryocytes. The lower of these has plentiful cytoplasm that is coarsely but indistinctly granulated with the pink anlage of platelets. The largest cell (lower left) is a fully mature megakaryocyte displaying at least 16 lobes. This elderly cell has shed its platelets, a process that occurs explosively on completion of maturation, hastened in this instance by the demands of severe thrombocytopenia. Several thousand platelets emanate from each spent megakaryocyte. Some are released while still aggregated, as may have been the case with the large mass of platelets at the bottom of **Figure 5-1,** but most are spun out in streamers from the collapsing walls of the ripened megakaryocyte. Some smaller megakaryocytes or megakaryocyte fragments enter the venous circulation and then lodge in pulmonary arterioles, from which locale they later dispatch their cargo of platelets.

Figures 5-3 and **5-4** (both ×2,000) portray an assortment of cell types often troublesome to nonveteran viewers, partly because these cells are fickle in their staining properties. At the upper right and center left of **Figure 5-3** are a pair of *eosinophil myelocytes*. Despite their ostentatious, glittering granules, these cells can be camouflaged or obscured by the slightest aberration in the staining process. In mature eosinophils as well as in eosinophil myelocytes, deviations in the pH may cause the granules to appear yellow, gray, or colorless. Conversely, in young eosinophil myelocytes the many dark blue primary granules may stand out so strongly that the cells are mistaken for promyelocytes or neutrophil myelocytes. At the top center is a neutrophil myelocyte that, despite its large nucleolus, is nearing maturity as signified by the copious cytoplasm and dearth of primary granules. At lower right is a neutrophil precursor that, all criteria considered, could be identified equally well as a mature promyelocyte or an immature myelocyte. Even in the best areas of the best-prepared marrow smear, about 5 to 10% of the cells are so altered by artifacts of preparation as to thwart identification. **Figure 5-3**, for example, displays at least 3 cells whose identities can only be surmised, and 2 cells are represented only by naked, smudged nuclei. The blurred, bluish *plasma cell* toward the upper right should be compared with 2 prototype plasma cells in **Figure 5-4**. These cells exhibit perfectly the peculiar coloration of plasma cell cytoplasm which, once appreciated, is unmistakable. This color is the muddy, opaque product of an unequal admixture of 2 complementary hues. The dominant ribosomal blue is partially grayed by the light pink of secretory immunoglobulin, particularly in the Golgi region centroidal from the eccentric nuclei. The special characteristics of plasma cells warrant reprise. Mature plasma cells are moderately large, usually from 14 to 18 μm across. Their cytoplasm is unusually copious for a cell having a nucleus as small as that of small lymphocytes. Eccentric placement of the nucleus is customary, and the dark purple chunks of condensed nuclear chromatin are more discrete and sharply defined than in lymphocytes. The blue-gray cytoplasm of plasma cells, which occupies about 80% of the cell, almost always contains vacuoles; most of these are small, blurred, and faintly tawny or pink, but some are large and clear, reflecting obstipation of endoplasmic secretory channels.

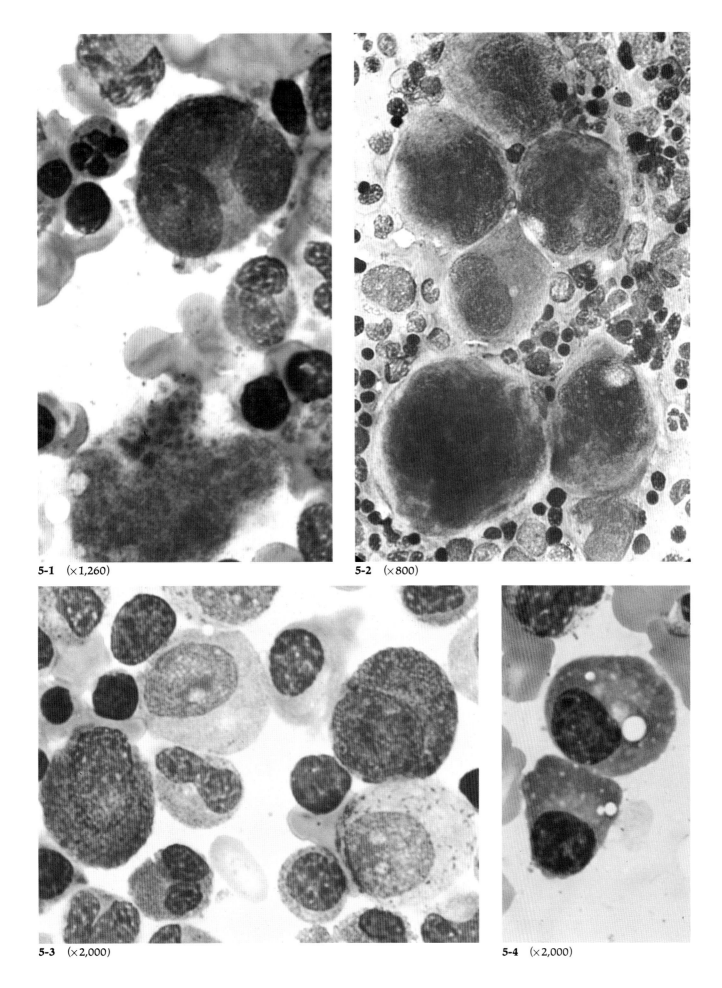

5-1 (×1,260)

5-2 (×800)

5-3 (×2,000)

5-4 (×2,000)

Normal Blood Cells

Figure 6. Cells of Blood

Numerically, the predominant cell of blood is the *red cell* (red blood cell, erythrocyte, rubricyte). **Figures 6-1** through **6-8** (all ×2,000) reveal the range of color variation considered acceptable. **Figures 6-7** and **6-8** show the very short rouleaux seen on a properly spread normal smear. The concentration of *platelets* can be estimated grossly by scanning the blood smear. An overabundance of platelets is usually discernible when the numbers exceed about 400,000/μl. Thrombocytopenia should be suspected when unclumped platelets are present in fewer than 1 high-dry field in 10. Finding few platelets on extensive scanning indicates platelet levels below 20,000 per μl, and encountering none signifies severe, potentially hazardous, thrombocytopenia.

A characteristic mature *neutrophil* is shown in **Figure 6-1**. Neutrophils ("polys") are remarkably uniform in size (diameter, 13 ± 1 μm) and possess 3 distinct nuclear segments, or lobes, connected in series by thin chromatin strands. Neutrophils are the infantry of host defense, the first cells to arrive at sites of pyogenic infections. While patrolling blood and barrier tissues, these brave but expendable cells locate noxious intruders by sensing chemoattractant gradients. Their nuclear design enables neutrophils to insinuate themselves between the endothelial lining cells of capillaries and to home in on extravascular inflammatory sites. They crawl toward their quarry like agitated inchworms, repetitiously flinging broad sticky capes (lamellipods) forward and hiking up their rearparts. Neither the contortions of locomotion nor the degranulation and vacuolation that ensue during an encounter with alien cells are evident in the peaceful normal neutrophil of **Figure 6-1**. This cell type, representing more than half of all leukocytes, possesses a faintly pink cytoplasm freckled with minute specific granulations. There are also about a dozen indistinct remnants of primary granules, seen as blurred purple smudges. Most of the dark purple chromatin is condensed along the margins of the segmented nucleus, and the rest is deposited in chunks. Neutrophil nuclei undergo various deformations as blood is smeared. The lobes may be overlapped, partly concealed, or disjoined. A few neutrophils have 4 nuclear segments, and fewer still have 5. In normal females, 2 to 3% of neutrophils have a unique rounded appendage of condensed sex chromatin known as the *drumstick*, or *Barr body*. The drumstick, 1.5 μm across, is connected to the inner aspect of a terminal lobe by a thin chromatin strand. About 5% of circulating neutrophils are unsegmented band forms, or *bands* (**Figure 6-2**), sometimes (cryptically) called *stabs*. These immediate precursors of neutrophils resemble them in size, cytoplasmic color, and degree of chromatin condensation. They differ in that the primary (azurophilic) granules of bands are more prominent and the nucleus is unsegmented, having a sausage shape that often is bent horseshoe-fashion.

Mature *eosinophils*, which constitute 5 to 10% of granulocytes, are identical in size to neutrophils. Their brilliant orange or red-orange refractile granules (**Figure 6-3**) identify them with certainty. These large, peroxidase-rich, specific granules are usually so numerous that the faintly pink background color is obscured. Even if relieved of granules, eosinophils could be identified by their unique nuclear segmentation. Although some eosinophils possess three nuclear lobes, 80% have two large round or potato-shaped lobes containing very heavily condensed chromatin.

Basophils (**Figure 6-4**) descend from the stem cell line common to all granulocytes, and their myeloblastic and promyelocytic precursors are indistinguishable from those of neutrophils and eosinophils. They account for barely one blood granulocyte in a thousand. The huge metachromatic (purple-black) specific granules are rich in histamine, serotonin, and leukotrienes. Although less numerous than the orange granules of eosinophils, basophil granules are sufficient in number and size to conceal most of the briochelike nucleus.

Lymphocytes, which are responsible for immunity, represent about one-third of blood leukocytes. Most lymphocytes contain a compact rounded or gently notched nucleus so uniform in size (9 μm across) as to provide a microyardstick for sizing nearby cells. The DNA of small lymphocytes is packed tightly into dense purple chromatin clumps enclosed by a scant cerulean veil of clear agranular cytoplasm (**Figures 6-7** and **6-8**). Approximately two-thirds of these inconspicuous cells are *T cells*, which participate in cell-mediated immune responses, and most of the remainder are *B cells*, lymphocytes genetically prepared to produce antibodies. T cells and B cells cannot be distinguished by light microscopy. About 10% of lymphocytes are large granular lymphocytes known as *natural killer cells* (**Figure 6-5**). NK cells possess abundant pale cytoplasm containing 10 to 20 reddish (azurophilic) granules, which when discharged upon virus-infected or HLA-incompatible target cells, create lethal large-hole hits. Often misnamed *atypical lymphocytes* because of their copious cytoplasm and large oblong nuclei, NK cells are xenophobic but normal cellular contributors to host resistance.

Several *monocytes*, which constitute 3 to 8% of blood leukocytes, are depicted in **Figures 6-6** through **6-8**. Monocytes, the largest blood cells, are round, measure 15 to 16 μm across, and have indented, often folded, nuclei. The nucleus—always corpulent, often kidney-shaped, and occupying about half the cell volume—has a loose, lacy network of chromatin strands. The reddish purple chromatin clumps are scattered throughout the nucleus and along the inner aspect of the nuclear membrane. There is no perinuclear halo. The ample cytoplasm is gray-blue and variably decorated with both fine and bold granules that are peroxidase positive.

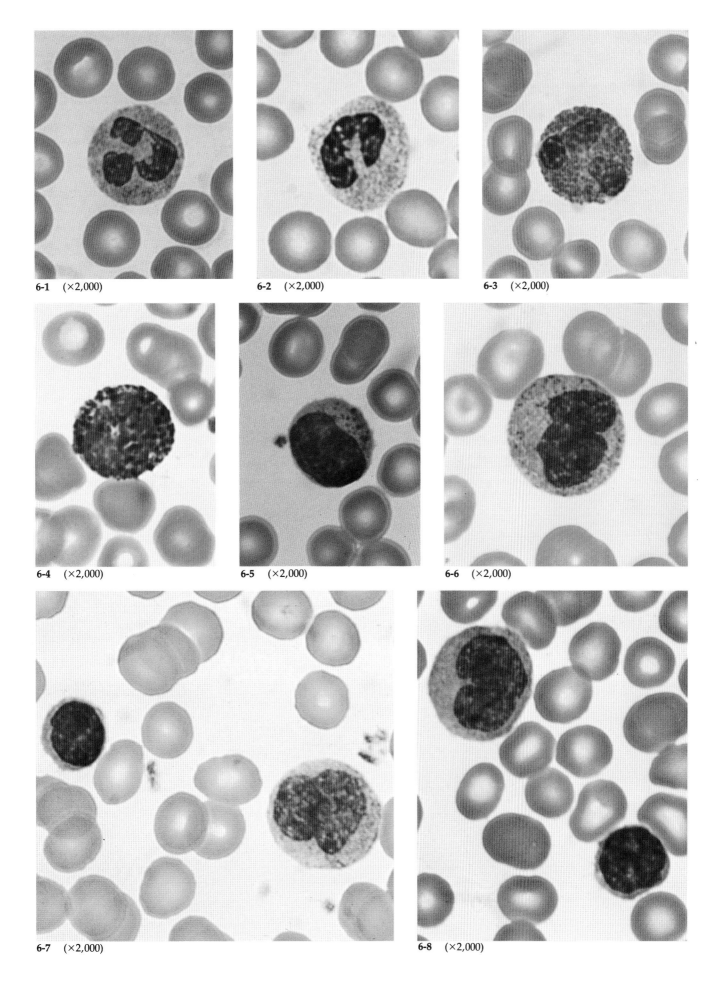

6-1 (×2,000)

6-2 (×2,000)

6-3 (×2,000)

6-4 (×2,000)

6-5 (×2,000)

6-6 (×2,000)

6-7 (×2,000)

6-8 (×2,000)

Intermission

Figure 7. A Morphologic Bestiary

Figures 7-1 through **7-6** present a pastiche of shockers, each guaranteed to freeze eye movement momentarily. From this collage of the outré, it is essential to distinguish friend from foe.

At the top of the page are 2 fearsome but friendly cell types—antithetical in function and different in provenance—that occasionally are dislodged during puncture of bone by a biopsy needle. **Figure 7-1** (×1,260) displays a characteristically huge, multinuclear *osteoclast*, torn from its endosteal moorings by the invading needle. These immense cells, ranging from 20 to 150 μm across, possess copious lightly basophilic cytoplasm, variably freckled by reddish lysosomal granules, which when abundant (as in the lower region of this cell) impart an eosinophilic cast. Their multiple (2 to 50), evenly spaced, rounded nuclei distinguish them from the vaguely similar but polylobated megakaryocytes and from the Langhans giant cells of chronic inflammation, in which nuclei are palisaded in arcuate array. Osteoclasts are physiologic multinucleated giant cells formed by fusion of precursor cells descended from monocytes. They are responsible for bone resorption under the opposing instructions of parathormone and calcitonin. Nestled against inner surfaces of bone, they exude acid hydrolases that excavate their own image in intaglio. Remodeling and creation of new bone is the task of *osteoblasts*, shown in **Figure 7-2** (×1,260). Descendants of fibroblasts, osteoblasts, when dislodged into marrow samples, form clusters of mottled, basophilic cells with eccentric nuclei that bear an unnerving resemblance to malignant plasma cells. The cytoplasm is webby rather than having the opaque look of plasma cells, and the cells are lacking in clear Golgi regions and secretory vacuoles. It is nevertheless important and reassuring to scan other fields, for osteoblasts are rarely found in more than a single cluster.

As evident in **Figure 7-3** (×800) the presence in blood of *epithelial cells*, singly or in small groups, is always startling but seldom misleading. These large pastel blue cells with abundant translucent cytoplasm and single pyknotic nuclei appear (and are) somnolent and friendly. They are thrust into the blood sample during skin puncture.

Within limits, marrow macrophages may engage in *erythrophagocytosis*, particularly when red cells or erythroblasts are dead or dying in large numbers from unbalanced ("ineffective") growth, as in megaloblastic anemia with intramedullary hemolysis. Normally marrow macrophages do not participate in the sort of feeding frenzy demonstrated in **Figure 7-4** (×1,260), even during the red cell slaughter associated with immune hemolytic anemias. The finding that phagocytosis is so wanton and promiscuous as to include host platelets or neutrophils as well as erythroid cells is suggestive of the outraged and unfocused immune response aroused by certain neoplasms. In this marrow, infiltrated elsewhere by T cell lymphoma cells, the resident macrophages were driven by the offended T cell network to extremes of gulosity. The macrophage in **Figure 7-4** appears benign (small, round, condensed nucleus and copious pale cytoplasm) but has glutted itself to the point of obstipation with red cells, platelets, and nucleated red cells, composting these with the ghostly remains of earlier victims. Comparable degrees of indiscriminate *hematophagocytosis* can also be seen in true histiocytic lymphoma and malignant histiocytosis, but in those rare disorders of macrophages the omnivores are the autocrine-driven tumor cells themselves. Malignant macrophages are recognizable by their deep blue cytoplasm and large, indented, uncondensed nuclei bearing emphatic nucleoli. A normal and more placid macrophage simply performing its housekeeping chores is shown in **Figure 7-5** (×2,000). Surrounded by promyelocytes (in this patient with acute promyelocytic leukemia), the macrophage has ingested and packaged granules of *hemosiderin* (hematoidin), the refuse of red cell precursors felled by leukemic infiltration. Hemosiderin ordinarily appears on Wright-Giemsa staining as chunks of green but, when admixed with red granules released by myeloid cells such as promyelocytes, deposits of the complementary pigments appear gray.

Advent of the AIDS era has introduced a common artifact to blood and marrow preparations, caused by spillage of talc during mandatory use of disposable gloves. At first glance, the pale blue umbilicated bodies at the center of **Figure 7-6** (×800) resemble storage macrophages. These are talc granules which, in their simulation of life, might be named *"exvitrocytes."*

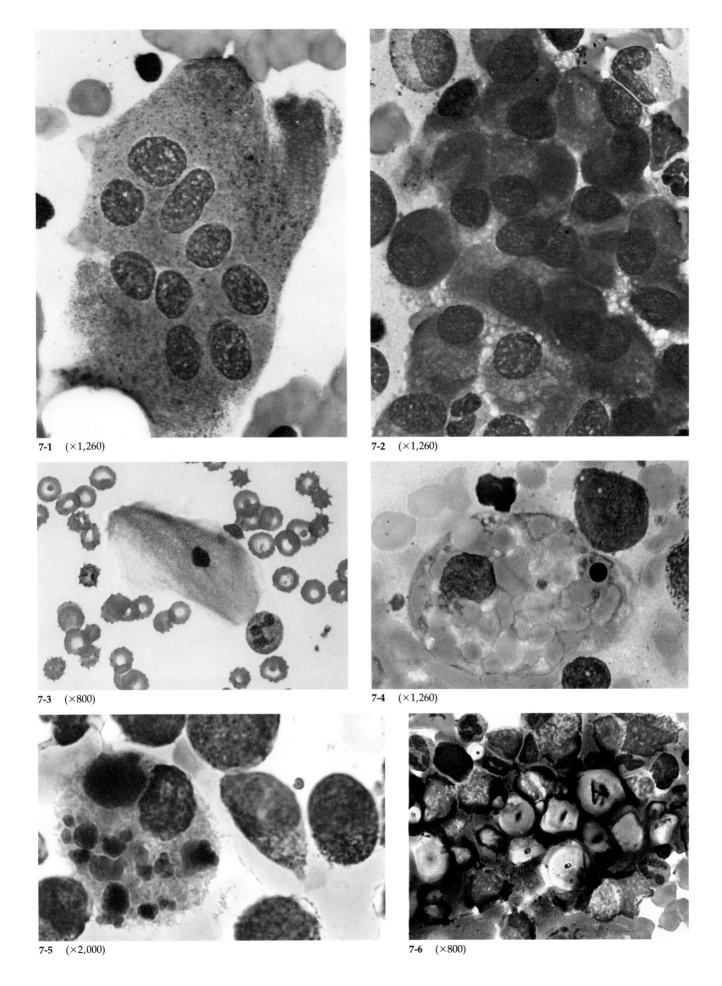

7-1　(×1,260)

7-2　(×1,260)

7-3　(×800)

7-4　(×1,260)

7-5　(×2,000)

7-6　(×800)

Bibliography

Bain BJ: Blood Cells. A Practical Guide. Philadelphia, JB Lippincott Company, 1989

Begemann H and Rastetter J: Atlas of Clinical Hematology, 4th ed. New York, Springer-Verlag, 1989

Boyde A et al: Optical and scanning electron microscopy in the single osteoclast resorption assay. Scan Electron Microsc 3 : 1259, 1985

Burns WA and Yook CR: Plastic sections and ultrastructural techniques in the evaluation of bone marrow pathology. Hematol Oncol Clin North Am 2 : 525, 1988

Cannistra SA and Griffin JD: Regulation of the production and function of granulocytes and monocytes. Semin Hematol 24 : 173, 1988

Casey TT et al: A simplified plastic embedding and immunohistologic technique for immunophenotypic analysis of human hematopoietic and lymphoid tissues. Am J Pathol 131 : 183, 1988

Chambers TJ: The pathobiology of the osteoclast. J Clin Pathol 38 : 241, 1985

Chambers TJ and Spector WG: Inflammatory giant cells. Immunobiology 161 : 283, 1982

Clarke PT et al: Differential white cell counting on the Coulter Counter. Clin Lab Haematol 7 : 335, 1985

Cooper MD: B lymphocytes. Normal development and function. N Engl J Med 317 : 1452, 1987

Dacie JV and Lewis SM: Practical Haematology, 7th ed. Edinburgh, Churchill Livingstone, 1991

Diggs LW et al: The Morphology of Human Blood Cells, 5th ed. Abbott Park, Ill, Abbott Laboratories, 1985

England JM and van Assendelft OW: Automated blood counters and their evaluation, in Automation and Quality Assurance in Haematology, Rowan RM and England JM, Eds. Oxford, Blackwell Scientific Publications, 1986

Frisch B and Bartl R: Atlas of Bone Marrow Pathology. Boston, Kluwer Academic Publishers, 1990

Glasser L and Fierderlein RL: Functional differentiation of normal human neutrophils. Blood 69 : 937, 1987

Hann IM et al: Colour Atlas of Paediatric Haematology. Oxford, Oxford University Press, 1983

Hayhoe FGJ and Quaglino D: Haematological Cytochemistry, 2nd ed. Edinburgh, Churchill Livingstone, 1988

Heckner F et al: Practical Microscopic Hematology, 3rd ed. Baltimore, Urban & Schwarzenberg, 1988

Henry JB, Ed: Clinical Diagnosis and Management by Laboratory Methods, 18th ed. Philadelphia, WB Saunders Company, 1991

Hillman RS and Finch CA: Red Cell Manual, 5th ed. Philadelphia, FA Davis Company, 1985

Hoffbrand AV and Pettit JE: Clinical Hematology Illustrated. An Integrated Text and Color Atlas. Philadelphia, WB Saunders Company, 1987

Hyun BH et al: Color Atlas of Clinical Hematology. New York, Igaku-Shoin Medical Publishers, 1986

Hyun BH, Ed: Bone Marrow Examination. Hematol Oncol Clin North Am 2 : 4, 1988

Johnston RB Jr: Monocytes and macrophages. N Engl J Med 318 : 747, 1988

Kjeldsberg C, Ed: Practical Diagnosis of Hematologic Disorders. Chicago, ASCP Press, 1989

Koepke JA, Ed: Laboratory Hematology. New York, Churchill Livingstone, 1984

McDonald GA et al: Atlas of Haematology, 5th ed. Edinburgh, Churchill Livingstone, 1988

McFarland W and Schecter GP: The lymphocyte in immunological reactions in vitro: ultrastructural studies. Blood 35 : 683, 1970

Murray GI: Is wax on the wane? J Pathol 156 : 187, 1988

Murray HW: Survival of intracellular pathogens within human mononuclear phagocytes. Semin Hematol 25 : 101, 1988

Nathan CF et al: Identification of interferon-γ as the lymphokine that activates human macrophage oxidative metabolism and antimicrobial activity. J Exp Med 158 : 670, 1983

Nathan CF: Secretory products of macrophages. J Clin Invest 79 : 319, 1987

Nelson L et al: Laboratory evaluation of the Coulter three-part electronic differential. Am J Clin Pathol 83 : 547, 1985

Plastic or paraffin? Editorial. Lancet 1 : 387, 1989

Rapaport SI: Introduction to Hematology, 2nd ed. Philadelphia, JB Lippincott Company, 1987

Rowan RM: ICSH recommendations for the analysis of red cell, white cell and platelet size distribution curves–Methods for fitting a single reference distribution and assessing its goodness of fit. Clin Lab Haematol 12 : 417, 1990

van Furth R: Current view on the mononuclear phagocyte system. Immunobiology 161 : 178, 1982

Zucker-Franklin D: Eosinophil function and disorders. Adv Intern Med 19 : 1, 1974

II. The Anemias

Megaloblastic Anemias

Figure 8. Megaloblastic Anemias: Blood

Thorough familiarity with the morphology of *megaloblastic anemias* is imperative, for these disorders are diagnosable and treatable. With rare exceptions, megaloblastic anemia responds completely either to parenteral cobalamin (vitamin B_{12}) or to folate. Two morphologic peculiarities are common to both deficiencies: (1) *Hypersegmentation* of neutrophil nuclei (**Figures 8-1,** ×800 and **8-5,** ×1,260) is an unmistakable logo of megaloblastic change and may presage anemia. The finding that any granulocytes have 6 or more nuclear segments, that more than 5% have 5 or more segments, or that the majority possess 4 or more segments signifies megaloblastic hypersegmentation. (2) As illustrated by **Figure 8-2** (×800), many red cells are large (macrocytes) and some are also egg-shaped *macro-ovalocytes.* Ovalocytes (egg-shaped cells), pathognomonic for megaloblastic anemia, should not be confused with elliptocytes. Both the redundant segmentation of neutrophils and the ovoid oblongation of red cells signify omission of 1 or more terminal divisions by marrow precursors. This kinetic lapse (maturation arrest) results from inability of proliferating marrow cells to garner the thymidylate needed for DNA replication and cell division in the absence of either essential cofactor—cobalamin or folate. Ordinarily, hypersegmentation and macro-ovalocytosis coexist. Indeed morphologic signs of maturation arrest, unbalanced growth, or nuclear-cytoplasmic asynchrony occur in many proliferating cell populations, including the epithelial cells of the tongue, small intestine, and uterus. Megaloblastic changes are not unique to blood and marrow cells; they are simply more obvious.

Figure 8-1 is a representative blood smear from a patient with pernicious anemia prior to parenteral cobalamin therapy. **Figure 8-2** portrays a comparably severe anemia caused by dietary deficiency of folate (folic acid, or pteroylglutamic acid). Both smears display extreme variations in cell size *(anisocytosis)* and shape *(poikilocytosis).* The majority of red cells are conspicuously macrocytic. Mingled with these are lesser numbers of odd-shaped cells about half-normal in size. Many macrocytes are round, but most are oblong, and some have the patented egg shape of the macro-ovalocyte. In the severely anemic patients represented in **Figures 8-1** and **8-2,** normal-appearing cells are almost totally replaced by a mixture of macrocytes, microcytes, and poikilocytes. Microcytes and poikilocytes are deformed in several stereotyped ways. Tapered or pear-shaped cells are often described collectively as *teardrop forms.* Some of the smallest cells are spherocytes, and a few in **Figure 8-2** are true *microspherocytes.* Very different in appearance from the teardrop forms and the microspherocytes are *fragmented forms* or *schistocytes,* examples of which are near the center of **Figure 8-2.** Although the survival of circulating red cells—the large, the small, and the misshapen—is curtailed moderately by splenic sequestration, the vast preponderance of cell slaughter occurs within the marrow, before the cells are released. The mean corpuscular volume (MCV) in megaloblastic anemia reflects the relative proportions of macrocytes and of cells of normal or diminished volumes, and, as anemia worsens, the diverse cell populations gravitate toward the extremes of size. If two-thirds of red cells are macrocytes of twice-normal volume, and one-third are half-normal in size, the MCV will be one and a half times normal, or approximately 140 μl. At the extreme upper left margin of **Figure 8-1** is a myelocyte, an immature myeloid cell that occasionally enters the circulation in severe megaloblastic anemias.

In response to worsening hypoxia, small numbers of nucleated red cells venture into the bloodstream. To the upper left of the small lymphocyte in **Figure 8-2** is a pathological orthochromatic erythroblast. This bizarre cell attests to the underappreciated fact that megaloblastic changes are most recognizable in the most mature erythroblasts. The nucleus is undergoing fragmentation (karyorrhexis). Some fragments are uncondensed, but 2 or 3 are pyknotic, spheroidal, and darkly purple: these nuclear remnants, when observed in an anucleate red cell, are termed *Howell-Jolly bodies.* **Figure 8-3** (×2,000) presents a closer view of Howell-Jolly bodies located in a macro-ovalocyte. Typically, they are purple-black, round or oblong, and 1 to 2 μm across. Red cells bearing Howell-Jolly bodies are prevalent in megaloblastic anemias and thalassemias; in patients without disturbed marrow, these inclusions are markers of splenic absence or hypofunction.

Numerically, the most severely and consistently depressed cells in megaloblastic anemias are the red cells, the numbers of which may decline below 1,000,000 per μl in untreated patients. Except in neglected, agonal cases, the white count seldom falls below 2,000 per μl. Platelet levels are invariably, but not predictably, depressed. Most platelet counts range from 50,000 to 150,000 per μl, but many are between 20,000 and 50,000, and some fall below 10,000 and incur risk of thrombocytopenic purpura. *Giant platelets* may appear in the blood as an expression of megaloblastic dysplasia of the marrow (**Figure 8-4,** ×2,000). Unlike its suitably small neighbor, this "megaplatelet" is nearly the size of a normal red cell.

Figure 8-5 underscores the significance of nuclear hypersegmentation in neutrophils as the most candid marker of megaloblastic arrest. Although several macrocytes are present in this field, these are not bona fide macro-ovalocytes and are outnumbered by normal and marginally aberrant forms. This equivocal melange might well be diagnosed as blood-loss anemia were it not for the pair of neutrophils possessing 7 or 8 lobes each.

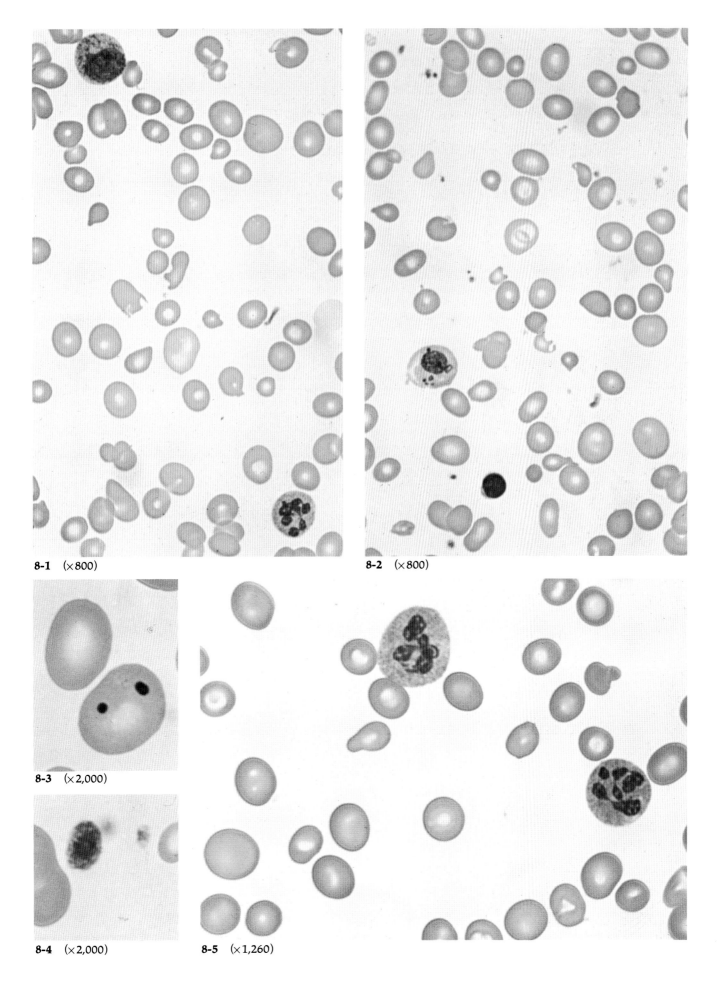

8-1 (×800)

8-2 (×800)

8-3 (×2,000)

8-4 (×2,000)

8-5 (×1,260)

Figure 9. Megaloblastic Marrow

Marrow abnormalities in established megaloblastic anemias are recognizable with a high-dry objective lens (**Figure 9-1**, ×800). These changes reflect an imbalance in the rate of maturation of the nucleus relative to that of cytoplasm. As cobalamin and folate act in series to generate thymidylate needed for DNA synthesis, deficiency of either vitamin slows nuclear replication and retards each step of maturation-division. As this retardation paves the way for uracil misincorporation, errors in DNA strand copying are cumulative with each division, and nuclear aberrations worsen progressively as maturation-division proceeds. In contrast, maturation of the cytoplasm and synthesis of hemoglobin are unimpaired. As a consequence of this imbalance between the rates of DNA synthesis by the nucleus and hemoglobin synthesis by cytoplasmic components, megaloblastic cells divide slowly and haltingly, but the size and hemoglobin content of the cells increase steadily. When DNA replication is frustrated, nuclear structure unravels. This is visible as uneven and erratic dispersion of the chromatin, with vacuolation. These changes occur to an equal extent in erythropoietic and myelopoietic cells but are easier to appreciate in the more stylized erythroid precursors. The coarse, dark-and-light speckling of megaloblastic chromatin creates a pattern like that of sliced salami. If DNA synthesis is suspended for several days, the cells die within the marrow, where they then are lysed or phagocytized. Intramedullary death and lysis of cells is often termed *ineffective erythropoiesis* or, more exactly, *ineffective hematopoiesis*. The few erythroblasts that reach the late orthochromatic stage usually are strikingly oversize, having cell volumes approaching twice normal, evidence of an omitted division step. Less publicized is the even more extraordinary macrocytosis exhibited by myeloid cells, particularly at the metamyelocyte and band stages. Presence of *giant metamyelocytes* and *giant bands* is possibly the most dependable single indication in the marrow of a megaloblastic process. Unbalanced growth also affects megakaryocytes, as indicated by pseudohyperploidy (hypersegmentation) in the marrow and by giant platelets in the blood. Spared from the cellular gigantism and nuclear-cytoplasmic asynchrony affecting marrow and epithelial cells are lymphocytes and plasma cells.

Apart from the 2 normal small lymphocytes, none of the 70-odd cells portrated in **Figure 9-1** is free of megaloblastic aberrations. In examining complex smears such as this, it helps to proceed in formulated or ritualistic steps. First, note the prevailing cellularity, which in this instance is considerable. Then scan cellular composition, noting that more than 15% of the cells are disruptued beyond recognition. Mark the presence of any exceptional or distracting cells, such as the erythroblast undergoing mitosis. Then systematically scrutinize each of the intact cells, proceeding clockwise. At this stage, one can make an initial assessment that the cells are predominately erythroblasts, that there are disproportionate numbers of basophilic and polychromatophilic erythroblasts, and that all erythroblasts at all stages are overtly megaloblastic. A second summary impression is that the myeloid series is represented by a mere half dozen granulocytes. Two of these—the largest cells in this field—are giant bands, with diameters in excess of 20 μm. After this initial scan, special attention may be given to selected cells. On comparing representative erythroid megaloblasts, proceeding in reverse order according to their apparent maturity, it becomes obvious that the most flagrantly megaloblastic cells are the most mature. The 2 proerythroblasts at the bottom right and the 1 in the far left–center are too young to display overt nuclear-cytoplasmic asynchrony, but the several pale, bloated, polychromatophilic erythroblasts at midfield show severely scrambled and wadded chromatin patterns. The observations above are confirmed at higher power in **Figure 9-2** (×1,260). The bright red-orange cytoplasmic granules of the eosinophil and heavy primary granules of the promyelocytes at the bottom and lower left are eye-catching, as always. Clockwise examination informs us that the upper area is populated by an enclave of erythroblasts with unevenly condensed, salami-like chromatin. Slightly lower down are two smaller but flagrant orthochromatic megaloblasts, the cytoplasm of one exhibiting a Howell-Jolly body. Despite the copious cytoplasm of these cells, their nuclei show only patchy condensation. Other salient findings in this field are the 2 giant bands at the upper left, a giant metamyelocyte at the upper right, and the hypersegmented (4-lobed) eosinophil.

The strangely beautiful patterns and colors of megaloblastic marrow cells are revealed in the grand Guignol tableau presented in **Figure 9-3** (×1,260). The proerythroblast at 7 o'clock is abnormal only in being slightly large, whereas the polychromatophilic and orthochromatic cells are gloriously grotesque. By comparing the giant band and the giant metamyelocyte (at 9 and 1 o'clock, respectively) with the polychromatophilic erythroblasts at 10 and 11 o'clock, one can see that in these representatives of 2 different cell lines the pattern of chromatin derangement is identical.

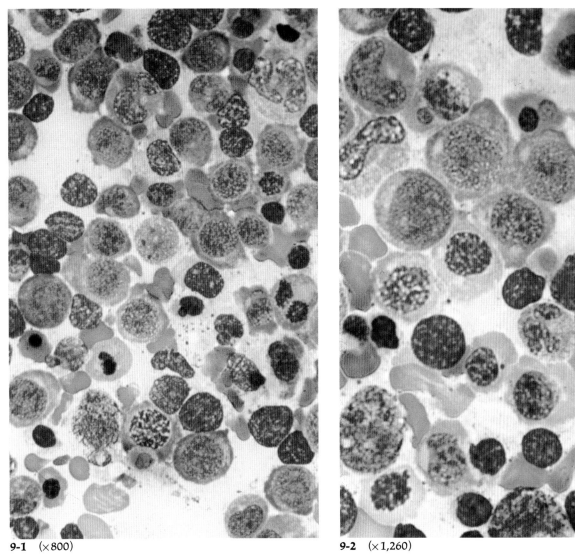

9-1 (×800)

9-2 (×1,260)

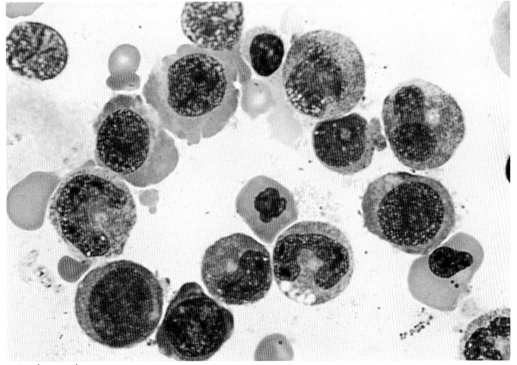

9-3 (×1,260)

Figure 10. Comparison of Normal and Megaloblastic Marrow. Influence of Complicating Hematosuppression.

Figure 10 is designed to recapitulate the salient differences between normal and megaloblastic marrows and to depict the confusing appearance of megaloblastic changes masked by hematosuppressive complications. **Figures 10-1** and **10-2** (both ×2,000) are juxtaposed vertically to facilitate comparisons between normal and megaloblastic erythroblasts. Similarly, **Figures 10-3** and **10-4** (both ×2,000) are aligned to highlight dissimilarities between normal and megaloblastic myeloid cells.

The normal basophilic erythroblast at the center of **Figure 10-1** displays emphatic chromatin aggregation, blue-purple nuclear metachromasia, and a perinuclear halo signifying nascent hemoglobin synthesis. Comparing this cell with surrounding polychromatophilic and orthochromatic cells provides an excellent exposition of the transitions characterizing normal erythroid maturation: stepwise reduction in cellular and nuclear size, darkening and coarsening of nuclear chromatin, and replacement of cytoplasmic basophilia by the bland eosinophilia of stained hemoglobin. (For a more lively hue, examine the glittering granules of the normal eosinophil to the right.) Their cytoplasm crammed with hemoglobin, 2 of the orthochromatic cells in **Figure 10-2** are more than 4 times larger than their normal counterparts, as can be appreciated by comparing them with the small lymphocytes in **Figures 10-3** and **10-4**. All cells in **Figure 10-2** display loss of synchrony between nuclear maturation and cytoplasmic accretion of hemoglobin. The cytoplasmic color of these cells and of the more basophilic cell at the top is patchy and variegated. The nuclear chromatin of all these megaloblasts is pale, juvenile, and in loose disarray.

Megaloblastic lesions in young myeloid cells also are more emphatic in later stages of differentiation. Metamyelocytes and bands may manifest extraordinary, often monstrous, changes. When the normal bands in **Figure 10-3** are compared with the cells in **Figure 10-4**, the gigantism of the megaloblastic metamyelocyte and 2 band forms is awesome. The band at the center, for example, exceeds 22 μm in diameter; in area it is 3 times normal and twice the size of the largest normal red cell precursors. These huge myeloid cells seldom appear in blood, presumably being too large to escape the marrow sinuses. The deranged appearance of chromatin in the 3 myeloid cells of **Figure 10-4** is indistinguishable from that of the comparably mature megaloblastic erythroblasts in **Figure 10-2**. Characteristic of megaloblastic marrow is the finding of many neutrophils with 4 or 5 nuclear segments. This seemingly modest deviation is sufficient to warrant a presumption of megaloblastosis.

Folate deficiency usually appears in the wake of debilitating processes such as malnutrition, chronic alcoholism, cirrhosis, or intestinal malabsorption, or during late pregnancy and the puerperium. Folate deficiency is endemic among the poor, elderly, reclusive, and alcoholic. As the result, the megaloblastic deformities of folate deficiency are commonly modified by other abnormalities. This is illustrated by marrow from an anemic patient with moderate folate deficiency complicated by chronic alcoholism plus pyogenic infection (**Figure 10-5**, ×1,260). This normally populated marrow lacks the striking erythroid predominance typical of uncomplicated megaloblastic anemia, and megaloblastic changes in both erythroid and myeloid cells are subdued and uneven. A clue that the hematopoietic response has been stifled by additional exogenous factors is the finding of sharply demarcated vacuoles in both the proerythroblast at lower right and an early promyelocyte at upper left. These small, clear intracytoplasmic inclusions vary only moderately in size, tend to occur in clusters, and occasionally pierce the nucleus. They are distinguished readily from the much larger spherical globules of fat shown in this field, for lipid droplets of lipocytes vary enormously in size and lie between cells. The most prevalent causes of vacuolation of erythroid or myeloid cells in marrow are infection, cytotoxic chemicals such as ethanol and agents used in chemotherapy, and idiosyncratic reactions to drugs such as chloramphenicol. During infection, particularly if pyogenic, myeloid cells are preferentially damaged and vacuoles tend to be fewer and larger. During hematosuppression by alcohol, cytoplasmic vacuoles are seen at all stages of erythroid differentiation, tending to be most pronounced in proerythroblasts. Vacuolation attributable to chloramphenicol suppression is restricted to proerythroblasts; indeed, in marrow displaying erythroid vacuolation induced by chloramphenicol, few erythroblasts mature beyond the proerythroblast stage. The riddled appearance of the young promyelocyte and the proerythroblast in **Figure 10-5** attests to the combined insults of intemperance and infection.

The miscellany of incidental findings in **Figure 10-5** variously corroborates the several diagnoses. Scattered through the field are a dozen or so round, olive green granules up to 1.5 μm in diameter. Dark olive or jade green granules on Wright-Giemsa smears almost always represent precipitated denatured hemoglobin and, consequently, occur in disorders marked by ineffective erythropoiesis and severe intramedullary hemolysis, particularly megaloblastic anemias and thalassemias. These chunky bodies are usually found as inclusions within phagocytic macrophages (also known in declining usage as *histiocytes*). Lying loose are many primary and secondary granules, a common finding in ineffective hematopoiesis. Finally, the increased background staining indicates hyperglobulinemia, in this case betokening the patient's cirrhosis.

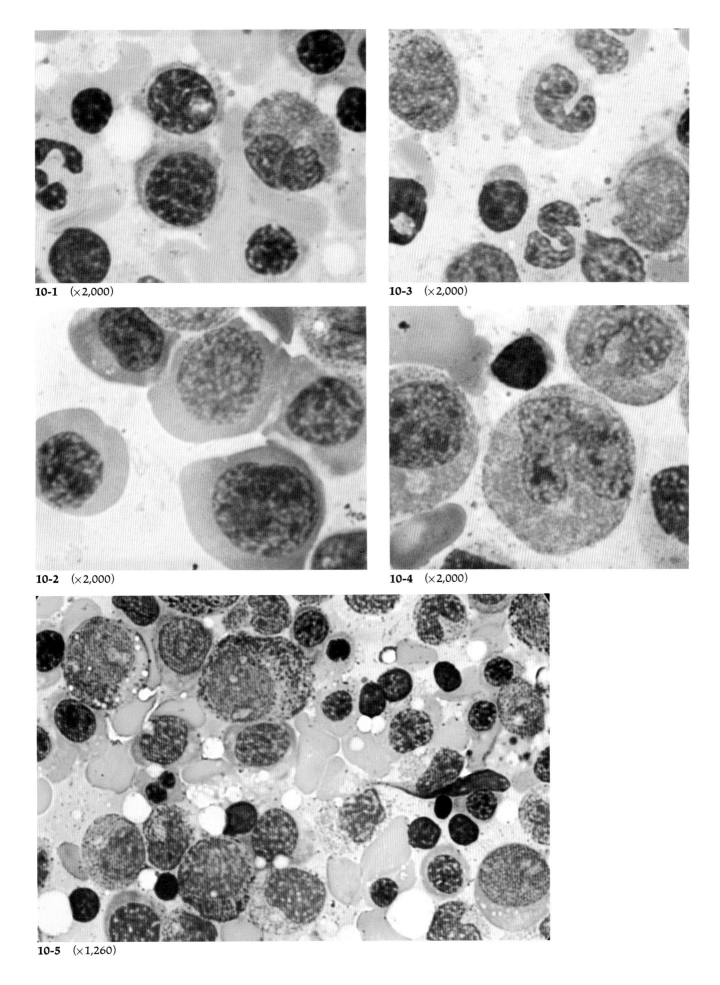

10-1 (×2,000)

10-3 (×2,000)

10-2 (×2,000)

10-4 (×2,000)

10-5 (×1,260)

Hypochromic Anemias

Figures 11 through 15. Introduction

The hypochromic anemias are distinguished by red cells that are deficient in hemoglobin. Hypochromic red cells are easily recognized by their washed-out appearance and broadened areas of central pallor. Hypochromia may also be defined and identified by determining the extent to which the mean cellular (corpuscular) hemoglobin (MCH) falls below the narrow range of normal, 30 ± 2 pg per cell. The pallor and paucity of the cytoplasm of maturing erythroblasts in the marrow attest to an underlying impairment of hemoglobin synthesis. In contrast, the anomalously high red cell count and increased numbers of erythropoietic cells in marrow affirm that the rate of red cell formation is undiminished. The several hypochromic disorders differ in causation, hematologic and clinical manifestations, and responsiveness to therapy. These dissimilarities, in turn, reflect the different steps in hemoglobin synthesis that are adversely affected. The most prevalent and the most treatable form of hypochromic anemia is caused by iron deficiency.

In addition to diminution in the red cell content of hemoglobin, the mean cellular (corpuscular) hemoglobin concentration (MCHC) is usually, but not invariably, reduced. Most hypochromic disorders also manifest microcytosis, as determined both by microscopy and by finding a low mean cellular (corpuscular) volume (MCV). In thalassemia, microcytosis is a salient feature, with MCV values falling between 50 and 75 fl per cell. In the acquired sideroblastic anemias and most pyridoxine-responsive anemias, the MCV may be normal, diminished, or increased, with about equal frequency. Only in uncomplicated iron deficiency anemia do hypochromia and microcytosis develop in tandem. Despite such differences, the several hypochromic entities are often cataloged generically as representing hypochromic microcytic anemias. Regardless of the inconstant association of hypochromia with microcytosis as determined by red cell indices, hypochromia and an increased area of central pallor of stained red cells are visible by light microscopy even when only a portion of the red cells is affected, as in iron deficiency of recent onset and most sideroblastic anemias. In thalassemias, hypochromia is often evident by microscopy despite a borderline or normal MCHC.

When the hemoglobin content of red cells is inadequate, secondary morphologic changes occur that are not specific but often assist in diagnosis. Their prominence depends on the etiology, degree of hypochromia, and severity of anemia. With mild or moderate hypochromia from any cause, target-like patterns are often evident in some cells. The term *target cell* alludes to the tinctorial pattern displayed by air-dried red cells wherein some hemoglobin is deposited in a centroidal smudge or puddle, separated by a variable clear zone from the hemoglobin of the peripheral rim. Target cells (*codocytes*, "Mexican hat" cells) having this bull's-eye staining pattern do not constitute a majority in hypochromic anemias as they do in certain unrelated, nonhypochromic disorders. Paradoxically, target forms may be least evident in the most severely hypochromic cells due to the extreme dearth of hemoglobin. Often, the pattern of hemoglobin deposition is poorly described by the word "target." The inner kernel of hemoglobin may be eccentric or it may bulge inward from the hemoglobin-stained periphery. There may be 2 or, rarely, 3 discrete "targets" in a single cell, especially in thin, hypochromic cells of large diameter or oblong shape. In some instances, a thin band of precipitated hemoglobin may span the cell.

Among the secondary changes in configuration affecting severely hypochromic red cells are conspicuous variations in size (anisocytosis) and in shape (poikilocytosis). Anisocytosis can be discovered and quantified through automated methods for assessing *red cell size distribution width* (RDW); RDWs generate histograms (population profiles), which are useful in sizing red cell subpopulations. Recognition of shape aberrations requires microscopy. The heterogeneity of size and shape among the cells in thalassemia major is unmatched. The red cells of iron deficiency anemia are not extensively or grotesquely misshapen unless anemia and hypochromia are exceptionally severe. Morphologic heterogeneity occurs in severely hypochromic red cells because each cell needs a certain minimum amount of hemoglobin simply as a structural requirement. When the MCH of red cells fails to reach about 20 pg, each cell lacks sufficient protein to attain the dimensions and rigidity essential for a normal shape. Consequently, these cells do not withstand well the "birth strain" of being squeezed forth through the marrow sinus walls and are damaged further by the trauma of being circulated, which in anemia is exacerbated by rapid and turbulent blood flow. A particular hazard occurs during repeated transit through the splenic red pulp. Within the marrow, if the erythroblasts have failed to accumulate an obligate quantity of hemoglobin, they are detained in marrow sinuses and may undergo an additional division, yielding abnormally small, end-stage cells. It is probable that an additional division accounts for those cases featuring extreme microcytosis, in which the MCV values are roughly half that of normal red cells. When the hemoglobin accrued is extremely low, erythroblasts fail to differentiate fully, cannot escape their native sinuses, and are destroyed within the marrow. This abortive intramedullary hemolysis, or *ineffective erythropoiesis*, is analogous to that in the megaloblastic anemias, despite basic differences in the pathogenesis and morphology of these 2 processes. The morphologic abnormalities of marrow erythroid cells in hypochromic anemias are graphic and diagnostic but not as obvious or picturesque as those in megaloblastic anemias.

Apart from iron deficiency, which may be the most common of all medical ailments, the several other similar-appearing anemias are sufficiently frequent and severe to warrant care in the differential diagnosis. This begins with blood cell morphology.

Figure 11. Iron Deficiency Anemia

Figure 11-1 (×800) shows a blood smear from a patient with severe *iron deficiency anemia.* Hypochromia is evident in nearly all red cells, which display expanded areas of central pallor. Usually, hypochromia is associated with microcytosis, recognizable by comparison with the nucleus of a small lymphocyte. Microcytosis is less obvious than hypochromia, however, for the average cell diameter is seldom diminished by more than 1 to 2 μm. Assorted aberrations in size and shape and in the pattern of hemoglobin distribution may be striking at blood hemoglobin levels below 5 or 6 g/dl, as shown here, although with mild anemia (**Figure 11-3,** ×1,260) morphologic changes are much less conspicuous. In most red cells of the severely anemic patient represented in **Figure 11-1,** hemoglobin is deposited unevenly in the peripheral rim. The subpopulations of pyknotic cells, elliptocytes, pale fragments, and etiolated target forms create pleomorphism, but this rarely rivals that of even mild thalassemia major. In iron deficiency, target cells are present in comparatively small numbers, regardless of the severity of anemia, and the few central puddles of hemoglobin are faint and smudged. Only occasional red cells resemble teardrops. Cells shaped like thick cigars—but often termed *pencil forms*—may be numerous in iron deficiency anemia, although none is present in this field. Several small cell fragments and a few shrunken, contracted forms are evident. Such forms appear only when anemia is severe. As illustrated in **Figure 11-1,** platelets often are overabundant in smears of iron-deficient blood, and the platelet count may be increased 2- to 4-fold. The findings in blood of nuclear hypersegmentation of neutrophils and in marrow of giant bands and metamyelocytes should arouse suspicion of a coexisting deficiency of folate or cobalamin. Unexplained mild hypersegmentation alone sometimes appears in uncomplicated protracted iron deficiency and may be a feature of the sideropenia itself. Significant by their absence from red cells in iron deficiency anemia are punctate basophilic stippling, Pappenheimer bodies, and siderotic granules.

The morphologic changes of marrow in iron deficiency are often overlooked because the erythroblasts are small and inconspicuous. At first glance, they resemble the artifactually shrunken cells that clutter up excessively thick smears of normal marrow. In **Figure 11-2** (×2,000), 8 erythroblasts are in full view. Their cytoplasm is so sparse, shaggy, and hemoglobin-poor as to be almost useless in judging the stage of cell maturation. Although none of these cells stains strongly for hemoglobin, 6 nuclei are in the orthochromatic stage. In 3 cells the chromatin is deep purple, and in 3 it is a darker blue-black, a heterochromatin hue unique to the closing stages of erythropoietic maturation. Iron-deficient erythroblasts are similar to lymphocytes in size and in their sparsity of cytoplasm, but the 2 lymphocytes in this field are distinguishable by their reddish purple chromatin. In addition, the chromatin clumps of lymphocytes are characteristically smeared and nonuniform in size. The darker chromatin masses in orthochromatic erythroblasts are more evenly dispersed, regular in size, and distinct. This often creates a cartwheel or checkered pattern, which on Wright-Giemsa staining is more definite than the chromatin motif of plasma cells. At each stage of maturation, iron-deficient erythroblasts are smaller than normal in both cytoplasmic and nuclear size. The nuclei of nearly all erythroblasts (about 95%) in iron deficiency marrow are in the last 2 stages of nuclear maturation. This represents a shift toward maturity, sometimes termed a *shift to the right.* Although young proerythroblasts are normal in number and appearance, basophilic and early polychromatophilic erythroblasts are scarce. Presumably, the transit (maturation) times for these early stages are rapid, whereas maturation thereafter is progressively slowed by a failure to amass sufficient hemoglobin. Accordingly, defective late-stage cells pile up, and many of them die unrequited within the marrow. The cytoplasm becomes increasingly shaggy as nuclear maturation proceeds. In all erythroblasts in this field, the scant cytoplasm stains very unevenly for blue, and hemoglobin coloration is barely discernible. In several cells, it is loculated in buff-colored areas adjacent to the nucleus, creating an irregular, often discontinuous, perinuclear zone. Not even in cells with condensed, nearly black, nuclei (late orthochromatic erythroblasts, or normoblasts) does hemoglobin-containing cytoplasm surround the nucleus.

Because mild iron deficiency anemia is exceedingly prevalent, is curable, and is commonly the first indication of gastrointestinal bleeding, it is important to recognize iron deficiency changes early, as exhibited in **Figure 11-3.** Juxtaposed in **Figure 11-4** (×1,260) is a normal blood smear. Variation in size and shape in mild iron deficiency is increased only slightly. Hypochromia and increased central pallor, the most consistent aberrations, affect the majority of cells, but very few cells display frank targeting. Microcytosis, a less constant feature of iron deficiency anemia than hypochromia, is also a less obvious one, as exemplified by this field. As compared with the normal red cells of **Figure 11-4,** roughly one-third of those in **Figure 11-3** appear undersized. The majority look normal despite the low MCV, and some pale cells have an expanded diameter. Note the significant increase in elliptical cells and a single contracted pyknocyte.

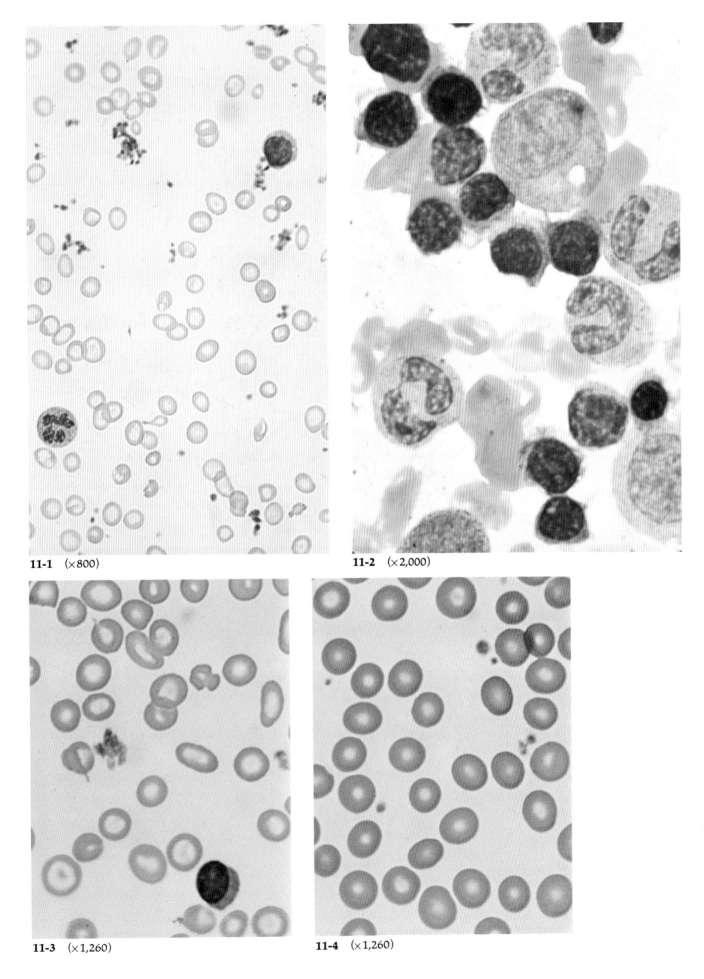

11-1 (×800)

11-2 (×2,000)

11-3 (×1,260)

11-4 (×1,260)

Figure 12. The Thalassemias. Thalassemia Minor versus Iron Deficiency.

Figures 12-2 and **12-3** portray the blood morphology of β *thalassemia minor*. Because exclusion of iron deficiency is an essential step in establishing diagnosis of this heterozygous or "trait" form of thalassemia, morphologic changes in mild and severe iron deficiency anemia are presented in the lower pictures (**Figures 12-4** and **12-5**) for comparison.

Thalassemias are hereditary hypochromic anemias caused by impaired synthesis of either the α or β chains of hemoglobin A ($\alpha_2\beta_2$). The α globin complex resides on the short arm of chromosome 16 and contains 2 α globin genes. Hence the 4 basic α thalassemia (*α-thal*) syndromes correspond to deletions or mutations of 1, 2, 3, or 4 α globin genes. A single deletion (α-thal-2) is harmless, double deletions cause thalassemia morphology with little or no anemia (α-thal-minor), triple deletions lead to chronic hemolytic anemia (hemoglobin H disease), and absence of all 4 α globin genes ordains death of erythroblasts in utero and hydrops fetalis. Inheritance of β thalassemia (*β-thal*) is more straightforward. As each chromosome 11 possesses only one β globin locus, members of affected families are either heterozygous and have microcytosis but little or no anemia (β-thal minor) or are homozygous (β-thal major); homozygotes develop severe hypochromic anemia because β chains are produced either in subnormal amounts (β^+-thal) or not at all (β^0-thal). Unbalanced synthesis of hemoglobin in either α or β thalassemia harms the erythron in 2 ways. Failure of α and β globin chains to match up equally to form the $\alpha_2\beta_2$ tetramers of hemoglobin reduces hemoglobinization of erythroblasts; either erythroblasts die in the marrow or, if their maturation is completed, the wretched red cells released into circulation are too small and deformed to survive well. Second, unmatched synthesis of α or β chains leads to their aggregation as Heinz body–like inclusions, which damage cells while in marrow or cause their later entrapment in the cruel crypts of splenic cords.

Figure 12-2 (×1,260) is characteristic of minimally expressed β thalassemia minor, in which there is striking uniform microcytosis associated incongruously with little or no anemia. A small minority of red cells is deformed, pyknotic, or targeted, but most appear normochromic. The impression of generalized microcytosis with relatively little hypochromia is borne out by red cell indices, which show low MCV values (range, 55 to 75 fl) but near-normal MCHCs. Dissociation of hypochromia from microcytosis is provisional evidence for thalassemia and against iron deficiency, but the finding of *punctate basophilic stippling* (**Figure 12-1**, ×2,000) is strongly supportive, for it unconditionally excludes iron deficiency. An easily overlooked marker of ineffective erythropoiesis, these fine blue-gray stipples evident on Wright-Giemsa stains represent clustered ribosomes. Pappenheimer bodies are larger, darker, and fewer, and siderotic granules require Prussian blue staining for iron.

In more severely expressed variants of thalassemia minor, most red cells possess some abnormality in addition to microcytosis (**Figure 12-3**, ×1,260). Target cells abound, poikilocytes are present along with stomatocytes, and blunt teardrop forms add to the general heterogeneity. The cell deformities found in patients with minimal or mild anemia due to β thalassemia minor are much more pronounced and varied than in comparably mild anemia due to iron deficiency. To facilitate morphologic comparison, blood smears from minimally expressed thalassemia minor (hemoglobin level, 12 to 15 g/dl) (**Figure 12-2**) and from a thalassemia variant associated with moderately ineffective erythropoiesis (hemoglobin level, 10 to 12 g/dl) (**Figure 12-3**) are aligned above smears from patients with mild anemia (**Figure 12-4**, ×1,260) and with severe anemia (**Figure 12-5**, ×1,260) caused by iron deficiency. With mild anemia, iron-deficient red cells display only slight anisocytosis, with no severely deformed cells and no distinct target forms. Many cells appear hypochromic, and most of these also have a reduced red cell diameter (compare red cells with the lymphocyte nucleus). In iron deficiency with hemoglobin levels below 5 to 6 g/dl (**Figure 12-5**), red cell pallor is so striking that the cells resemble wafers, and these pale, flattened discs are admixed with assorted poikilocytes, creating a chaotic pattern reminiscent of thalassemia minor. The hypochromia may be every bit as pronounced as in thalassemia major, but the degree of deformation does not match that of β-thal major, and targeting, a thalassemia signature, is inappreciable.

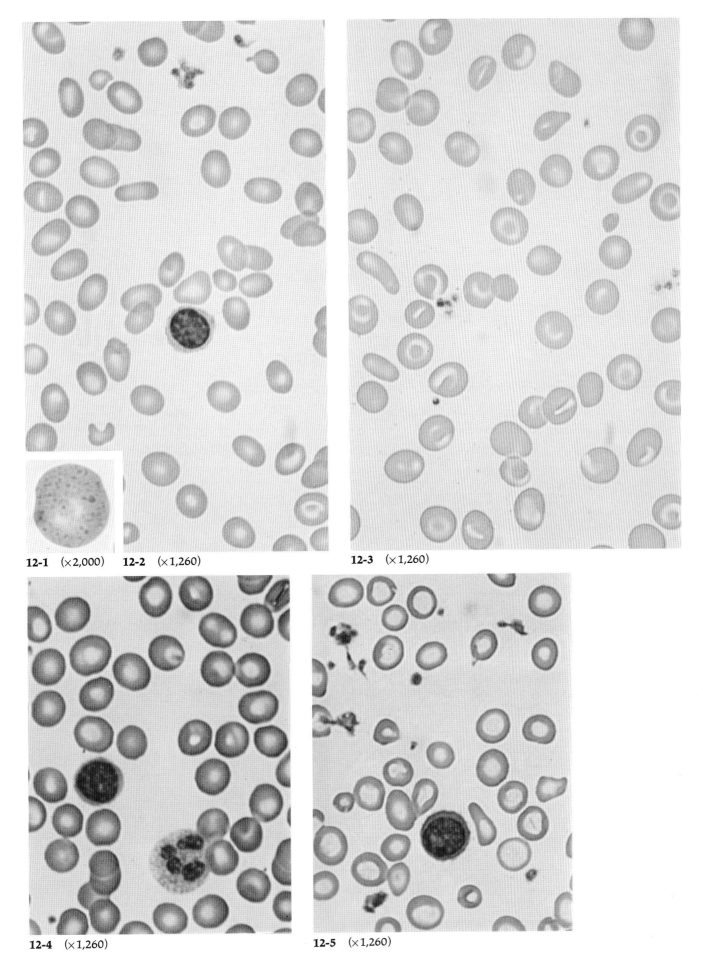

12-1 (×2,000)　**12-2** (×1,260)　　　**12-3** (×1,260)

12-4 (×1,260)　　　**12-5** (×1,260)

Figure 13. β Thalassemia Major. The α Thalassemia Syndromes.

In *β thalassemia major* (homozygous β-thal), anemia is severe and red cells display a grotesque, kaleidoscopic heterogeneity unrivaled among the anemias. Most cells are very small (MCV, 50 to 60 fl) and many are mere fragments, desperate products of reiterative divisions by the hurried marrow. Most numerous and illustrative of the inability of erythroblasts to accumulate adequate hemoglobin are the flattened forms with large areas of central pallor, thin pink rims, and a mad variety in shape (**Figure 13-1**, ×1,260). Many of these ghostly waferlike cells are broadened in their empty laxity like unfilled balloons, causing them to spread out abnormally during air drying, often leaving behind islands of hemoglobin that lend a targeted appearance. The cells are frail and readily deformed during circulation, causing many to become stretched and drawn out into tailed or *teardrop forms*. Almost as numerous are cells that appear to be cleaved in half or to have had a bite removed. "Bite-out" deformities are indicators that bulky inclusions had been forcibly torn from the cell. In the spleen, β-thal red cells loaded with α chain baggage are hung up in the slitlike defiles connecting cords to sinuses. This eventuates either in the arrest and destruction of the red cell or in a tugging affair, during which the cell may break free but in so doing either loses a "bite" or acquires a tail (teardrop shape) as a memento. Near the top of **Figure 13-1** is a cell with an exemplary bite-out deformity.

Figure 13-4 (×1,260) attests to a dramatic alteration in morphology of thalassemic cells that follows splenectomy: virtual disappearance of both teardrop forms and bite-out deformities. Splenectomy in thalassemia not only removes the stern chambers of the spleen but also leads to a set of morphologic alterations that collectively signify the spleenless state. Normally the spleen culls inclusions from imperfect young red cells, acts as a finishing school for prematurely released normoblasts, polishes surplus lipid from red cell membranes, and serves as a transit pool for platelets. Absence of spleen function is evidenced in **Figure 13-4** by the presence of dark granular Pappenheimer bodies in a red cell near the top, the legions of nucleated red cells, expansion of red cell membrane area and consequent targeting, and a surfeit of platelets.

Figure 13-2 (×1,260) portrays the uniform microcytosis, slight hypochromia, and moderate targeting found in *α thalassemia minor*. Absence of two α globin genes—either as a double deletion in cis (the α-thal-1 gene), which is prevalent in Asians, or as 2 single deletions in trans, as occurs commonly in individuals of black African descent—causes only modest accumulations of unmatched β chains. This inflicts limited damage to red cells, and erythropoiesis is only mildly ineffective. Among blacks, in whom the single deletion (α-thal-2) gene predominates, hemoglobin H disease is rare, whereas in Asian populations all α thalassemia syndromes are possible, including hydrops fetalis.

Hemoglobin H disease is caused by deletion or mutation of 3 of the 4 α globin genes and hence is most prevalent in Asians. Hemoglobin H disease is characterized by moderate hemolytic anemia, elevated reticulocyte levels, and hypochromic microcytic red cells displaying conspicuous targeting (**Figure 13-3**, ×1,260). This thalassemic disorder received its name from the injurious pileup within red cells of unpaired β chains, which arrange themselves as unstable tetramers ($β_4$). The $β_4$ tetramers of hemoglobin H, representing up to 30% of red cell hemoglobin, have a very high oxygen affinity and are useless in oxygen transport. In a portion of red cells, hemoglobin H can be precipitated readily in vitro by adding a redox dye such as brilliant cresyl blue (BCB). Spontaneous flocculation of these globin chains in vivo is not as extensive or injurious as that of α chains in β thalassemia, and bite-out deformities are inconspicuous.

Homozygous inheritance of α-thal-1, with absence of all 4 α genes, is incompatible with life. The predominant hemoglobin is *hemoglobin Bart's* ($γ_4$), which has an intolerably high oxygen affinity. The affected fetus develops hydrops fetalis and either is stillborn or expires within hours after birth. At delivery, cord blood contains a mixture of pyknocytes, polychromatophils, and erythroblasts at various levels of differentiation (**Figure 13-5**, ×1,260). This melancholy progression can be anticipated by demonstrating absence of α globin genes from fetal DNA obtained from amniotic fluid in suspect pregnancies.

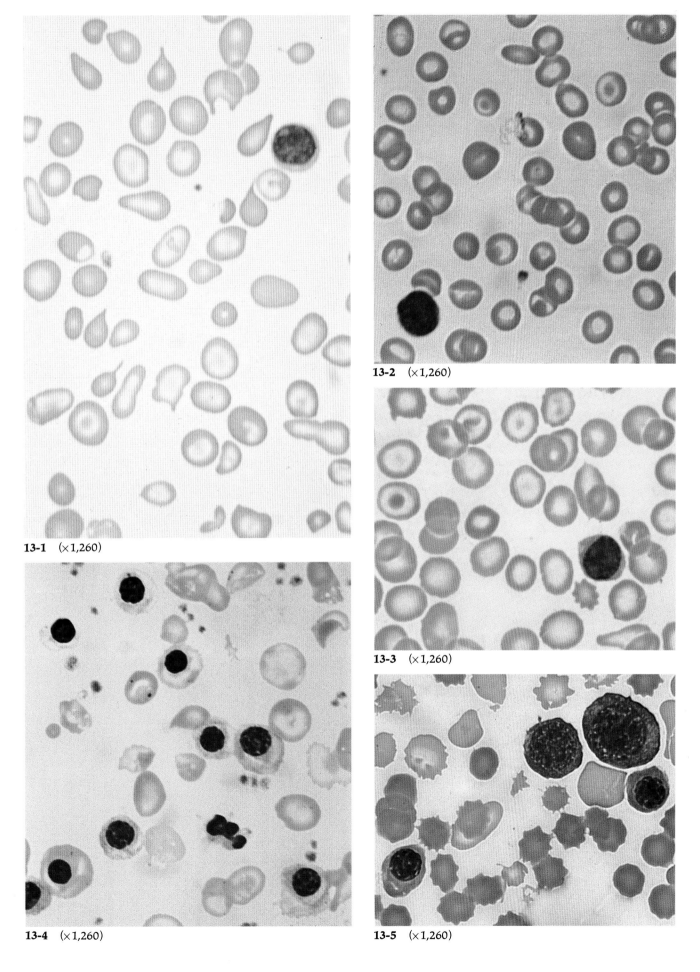

13-1　(×1,260)

13-2　(×1,260)

13-3　(×1,260)

13-4　(×1,260)

13-5　(×1,260)

Figure 14. Combined Hypochromic and Megaloblastic Anemia (Dimorphic Anemia). Assessment of Marrow Iron.

The basic defect of megaloblastic anemias is impairment in DNA synthesis, and that of hypochromic anemias is reduction in hemoglobin synthesis. When coincident, the 2 defects have opposing morphologic effects. If comparably severe, these two processes nullify each other in erythropoietic cells by restoring balance in the rates of nuclear and cytoplasmic differentiation. The megaloblastic changes in the myeloid series are not offset, however, as is illustrated by the hypersegmented neutrophils in **Figure 14-1** (×800). The expression *dimorphic anemia* understates the range of polymorphisms possible when megaloblastic anemia and iron deficiency anemia coexist. As is true also of certain sideroblastic anemias, anemia caused by the compounding of iron deficiency and either folate or cobalamin deficiency is usually marked by 3 rather than 2 subpopulations of red cells. **Figures 14-1** and **14-2** (both ×1,260) show the admixed abnormalities in the blood and marrow, respectively, of combined iron deficiency and folate deficiency. The dominant aberrations of red cells are hypochromia and microcytosis, affecting all but a few cells. Hypochromia can be recognized when the central pallor of a red cell appreciably exceeds 25% of its area (i.e., it spans more than half the cell diameter). The microcytosis in **Figure 14-1** might not be obvious without reference to the lymphocyte. The nucleus of this normal small lymphocyte is about 9 μm across; as this is 2 to 3 μm wider than the average diameter of the red cells shown, the impression of microcytosis is validated. As illustrated here, the hypochromic and microcytic cells of severe iron deficiency are usually associated with a minor population of poikilocytes and occasional teardrop forms. Suspicion that something additional is going on is raised by the sight of a single large macro-ovalocyte at midright. Proof that this implicates a covert megaloblastic disorder is provided by the 2 neutrophils, both of which exceed the limit in nuclear segmentation (about 6 segments each). Two features differentiate these from cells with "twinning" deformity: all segments are linked in series, and neither cell appears enlarged by twofold. The combination of macro-ovalocytes and hypersegmented neutrophils, however few their numbers, is decisive evidence of complicating megaloblastic change.

A marrow aspirate from the same patient (**Figure 14-2**) shows an increase in the proportion of erythropoietic cells, with an inverted myeloid:erythroid (M : E) ratio of 1 : 2. Most are polychromatophilic erythroblasts which, along with the several ragged orthochromatic erythroblasts, are deficient in cytoplasm and stain feebly or not at all for hemoglobin. Nuclear chromatin clumping in most erythroid cells is mildly irregular, suggesting minimal megaloblastic change. This impression is strengthened by the nuclear-cytoplasmic asynchrony of the young basophilic erythroblast at lower center. The nuclear chromatin pattern identifies this cell as a late proerythroblast, but an inappropriate cytoplasmic pinkness and polychromatophilia signify discordant maturation. The nucleated target cell at top right bears evidence of both deficiencies. It is oversized for a late orthochromatic erythroblast and very poor in hemoglobin. Among the myelopoietic cells, megaloblastoid changes are comparably modest.

The marrow samples portrayed in **Figure 14-3** (×2,000) and **14-4** (×800) demonstrate the appearance of excessive iron (hemosiderin and ferritin) stores. When unstained (**Figure 14-3**), marrow iron is seen as deep golden granules, some of which are aggregated into lumpy, refractile nuggets 5 to 10 μm across. Surplus iron as *hemosiderin* and *ferritin* is mainly packaged in lysosomes and stored in macrophages deployed amidst the stromal cells of marrow. In evaluating marrow aspirates for iron, one should examine thickly cellular areas of the fresh smear, where stromal components can be seen by the naked eye as whitish flecks. Iron stores of marrow cannot be assessed with certainty without use of the Prussian blue stain, which is sensitive, specific, and semiquantitative—assuming the marrow preparation contains a sufficient quantity of stromal cells. The marrow obtained by needle biopsy and depicted in **Figure 14-4** showed very little hemosiderin when unstained; after the film was stained by the Prussian blue reaction and then counterstained with the red dye safranin, the indigo blue masses and granules of stained hemosiderin stood out sharply. In areas where marrow cells are adequately spread out and the blue or blue-green aggregates are comparatively small, it is evident that the iron is deposited within stromal cells. That this patient had a sideroblastic anemia is attested to by *ringed sideroblasts* at the top left of the figure. The iron-staining reagent, Prussian blue (potassium ferrocyanide), spontaneously forms blue-black precipitates during exposure to air. If not removed from the reagent by filtration immediately prior to the staining procedure, these granular precipitates may deposit onto the coverslip. This artifact can be identified by the black, siltlike appearance of the deposits and their random deposition unrelated to the distribution of cells.

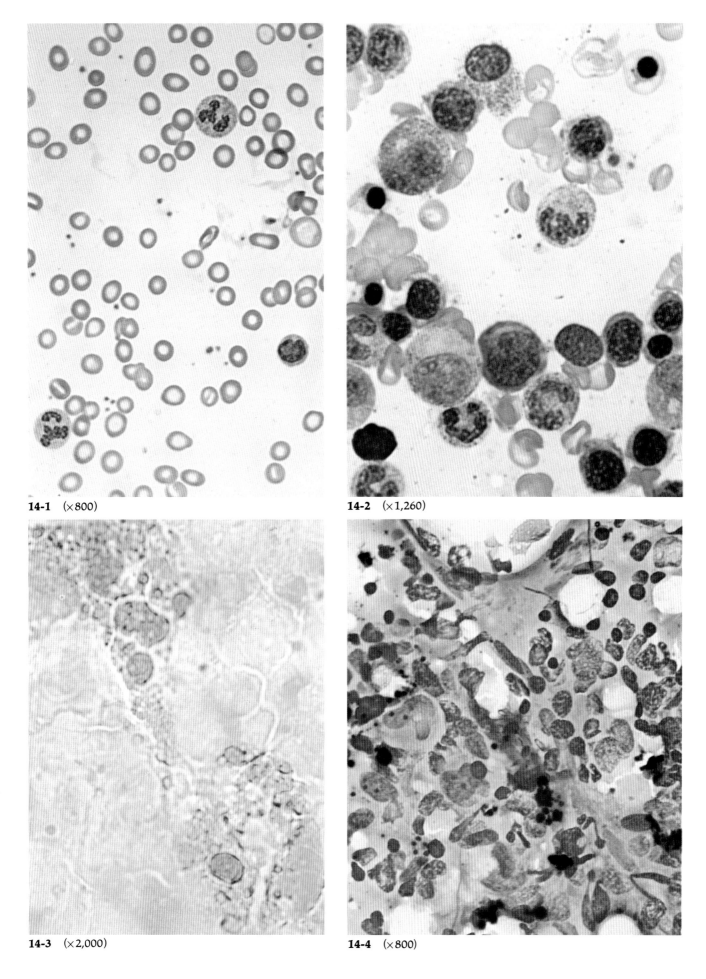

14-1　(×800)

14-2　(×1,260)

14-3　(×2,000)

14-4　(×800)

Figure 15. Sideroblastic Anemias

Figure 15 exhibits several sideroblastic abnormalities. All 6 pictures are enlarged ×2,000. **Figures 15-2, 15-5,** and **15-6** show smears stained with Prussian blue and counterstained with safranin; the remainder are stained with Wright-Giemsa.

Sideroblastic anemias are a diverse group of hypochromic microcytic disorders caused by defective iron utilization within erythropoietic cells. Failure in iron processing usually stems from a reduction in δ-aminolevulinic acid (ALA)-synthetase activity, the initial and rate-limiting step in heme biosynthesis. This malfunction not only deprives differentiating erythroblasts of sufficient hemoglobin but also causes toxic accumulations of iron in mitochondrial cristae, thereby also compromising the terminal steps of heme synthesis. Accumulations of iron slag in mitochondria are responsible for the morphologic insignia of sideroblastic anemias, *ringed sideroblasts*. The morphologic triad of sideroblastic anemias combines the following: hypochromic red cells with erythroid dimorphism, hyperferremia and increased tissue iron, and ringed sideroblasts. Three criteria must be met for authentication of ringed sideroblasts: (1) the iron-staining granules must be abnormally large, (2) their number should exceed 5 or 6, and (3) they must form an arc extending around at least one-third of the nucleus. When more than 10% of orthochromatic nuclei in marrow are hugged closely by a collar of large Prussian blue–staining granules (**Figure 15-6**), the diagnosis is made.

The underlying metabolic problem may be hereditary or acquired, most of the latter being idiopathic (primary) but some being secondary to known mitochondrial toxins such as lead and alcohol. In half of kindred with the hereditary disorder but in only 5% of those (usually elderly) individuals with idiopathic sideroblastic anemia, the anemia responds to large doses of pyridoxine, an obligate coenzyme for ALA synthesis. This has engendered the term *pyridoxine-responsive anemia*, although for sustained remission repeated pharmacologic doses are required and, even during response, hypochromia and microcytosis persist. Morphology of sideroblastic anemias is very confusing: microcytic red cells are commonly admixed with macrocytes, creating erythroid dimorphism. Megaloblastic changes may add to the complexity, responding unevenly to folate. About half of idiopathic cases have refractory marrow dysplasia with clonal chromosomal anomalies, and in about 10% of these patients the dysplastic marrow transforms eventually into acute myelogenous leukemia. Acquired *refractory anemia* with ringed sideroblasts is now incorporated among the *myelodysplastic syndromes* (see Figure 31).

Figure 15-1 portrays the blood of a house painter who developed severe anemia during heavy inhalational exposure to lead incurred as he removed lead paint by sanding. His anemia was a product of hemolysis plus marrow-cell injury with sideroblastic changes. Most red cells are hypochromic and microcytic, but the two largest cells are ovoid and show coarse *punctate basophilic stippling*. Coarse basophilic stippling, a notorious feature of lead poisoning, is limited to the youngest red cells, and thus only a small percentage of cells are heavily stippled.

Figure 15-2 depicts *siderotic granules* as they appear after staining with Prussian blue. The largest, most hypochromic cell contains 8 or 9 dark blue inclusions that are clustered at one side of the cell. Red cells with iron-stainable inclusions are termed *siderocytes*. Siderocytes are uncommon even in hyperferremic states but may appear in large numbers after splenectomy, along with other inclusions normally culled out by the spleen.

Figure 15-3 shows a blood smear from a patient with sideroblastic anemia and chronic alcoholism. Two cells contain inclusions visible on Wright-Giemsa stain. The polychromatophil at the upper right contains several irregular inclusions known as *Pappenheimer bodies*. Pappenheimer bodies are stained by Wright-Giemsa because they contain clumps of ribosomes (which stain blue) admixed with coprecipitated iron-rich mitochondria and ferritin. If stained for iron these siderotic inclusions would appear larger and bluer. The lower inclusion-containing cell contains both a dark purple Howell-Jolly body and a smaller blue-gray Pappenheimer body. In **Figure 15-4**, Pappenheimer bodies are present in 2 cells. The large, pale polychromatophilic target cell next to the monocyte is peppered with these inclusions, and several are visible in the small pale erythroblast.

In **Figures 15-5** and **15-6**, the marrow cells were obtained respectively from a patient with sideroblastic anemia attributed to chronic alcoholism and from a patient with refractory anemia. The smears were stained with Prussian blue. Both ringed sideroblasts in **Figure 15-5** are late orthochromatic cells. The large size, deep blue color, and close proximity to the nucleus of the siderotic granules mark the cells as pathological even though the granules do not form a long arc. In **Figure 15-6**, 5 cells are heavily laden with iron inclusions and all meet the 3 criteria for ringed sideroblasts.

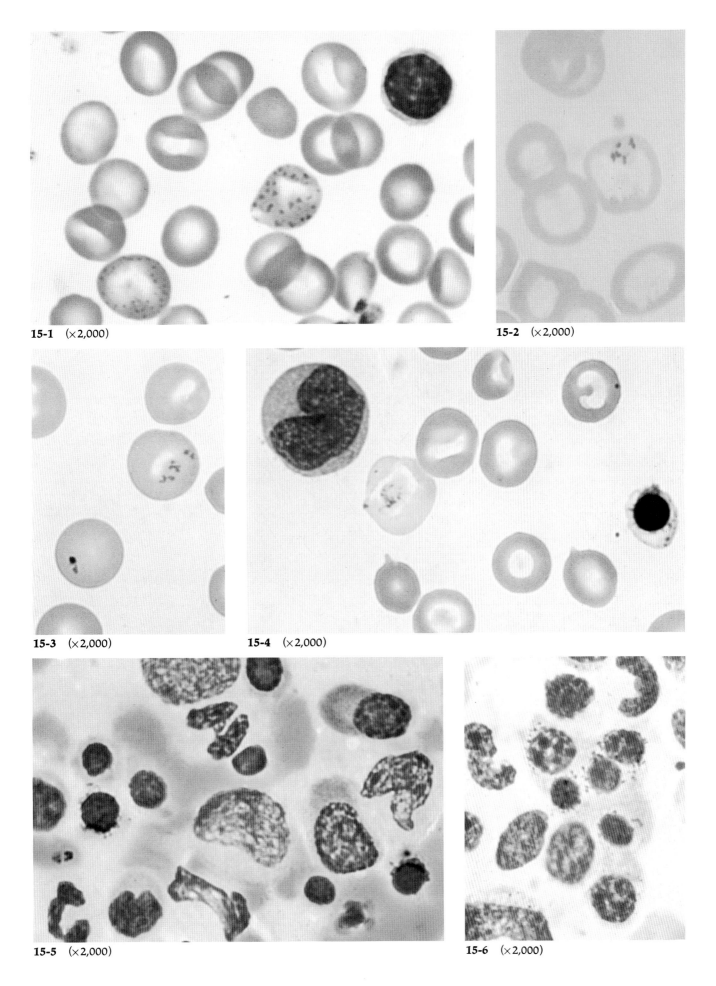

15-1 (×2,000)

15-2 (×2,000)

15-3 (×2,000)

15-4 (×2,000)

15-5 (×2,000)

15-6 (×2,000)

Hemolytic Anemias

Figures 16 through 25. Introduction

Hemolytic anemias are defined by 2 characteristics: (1) an increased rate of destruction *(hemolysis)* of circulating red cells and (2) an increased rate of erythropoiesis. In the vast majority of hemolytic diseases, hemolysis is caused by random destruction rather than by accelerated senescence. Rarely, red cells are dissolved while in circulation *(intravascular hemolysis)*, but in most hemolytic processes destruction is initiated or concluded by trapping of cells in the sinuses of the spleen or liver, a process ineptly termed *extravascular hemolysis*. Most anemias have a hemolytic component, but for practical purposes disorders in which hemolysis occurs principally during circulation should be segregated from processes such as thalassemia that are dominated by intramedullary hemolysis. Most hemolytic anemias stemming from defects intrinsic to red cells are hereditary, and virtually all forms of hemolysis originating extrinsic to the red cell are acquired.

Laboratory findings typical of established hemolytic anemias are: elevated reticulocyte levels and hyperplasia of erythropoietic marrow cells; elevated serum levels of indirect-reacting bilirubin (usually); a rise in plasma hemoglobin concentration (frequently); lowering or depletion of serum haptoglobin (almost always); hemosiderinuria (frequently), sometimes attended by hemoglobinuria; increased numbers of spherocytes in the peripheral blood (almost always); and "spontaneous" lysis of red cells during routine laboratory handling (commonly). In addition, urobilinogen excretion is increased, and the serum level of lactic acid dehydrogenase (LDH) may rise to several times normal.

The rare disorder *paroxysmal nocturnal hemoglobinuria* (PNH) provides exceptions to the generalizations just made. Spherocytosis, a feature of most hemolytic processes, is not present, and serum bilirubin is elevated little, if at all. Indeed, the red cells in PNH are singularly free of morphologic abnormalities. In contrast, the plasma level of hemoglobin in PNH is conspicuously increased, as is the level of a derivative brown pigment, methemalbumin. Together the 2 heme proteins give the plasma a mahogany color. Hemosiderinuria persists, whereas hemoglobinuria is inconstant.

Characteristic clues to hemolytic anemia are unexplained reduction or decline in hemoglobin concentration and reticulocytosis that persists without benefiting the hemoglobin level. In chronic hemolytic disorders, the erythropoietic response is often sufficiently vigorous to offset the heightened rate of red cell destruction. This erythropoietic adjustment, termed *compensated hemolytic anemia*, may entail mild jaundice. Although elevated reticulocyte levels are almost constant in hemolytic disorders, intercurrent infections, uremia, medications, or other causes of marrow suppression may induce spells of reticulocytopenia.

Bear in mind that 1 or more prime indicators of hemolytic anemia may, for a time, be suspended because of abolition of the compensatory response by hematosuppressive factors. The onset of infection, however mild, may cause virtual disappearance of reticulocytes. In severe hemolytic processes, the combination of hemolysis and myelosuppression may convert a controlled anemic disorder into a precipitous, life-threatening one. A more insidious hematosuppression may result from complicating uremia or the increased folate needed by hyperproliferative marrow. Relative deficiency of folate may ensue without obvious morphologic evidence of folate deficiency. If the hemolytic process is moderate, as in mild cases of hereditary spherocytosis (HS), the diagnosis may be missed throughout early life. In a woman with subclinical HS, the heightened requirement for folate during and after pregnancy, by deepening the deficit constantly imposed by HS alone, may induce a megaloblastic anemia commencing late in pregnancy, the kind mislabeled *pernicious anemia of pregnancy*. This potentially hazardous complication can be corrected by administering folate; only then may spherocytosis and other laboratory stigmata of underlying HS emerge.

The most important of the acquired hemolytic anemias fall into 8 major categories. (1) *Microangiopathic hemolytic anemias* arise as complications of processes that affect the microvasculature or create turbulent left ventricular outflow. (2) *Immunohemolytic anemias* are acquired disorders often called *autoimmune hemolytic anemias* in jargon, because antibodies react with self antigens. (3) The diverse and unrelated hemolytic entities—*spur cell anemia, acanthocytosis,* and *PNH*—result from alterations in the structure, contours, and surface properties of the red cell membrane. (4) Genetic hemolytic processes that affect the skeletal structure or permeability of the cell membrane include *HS, hereditary elliptocytosis, hereditary stomatocytosis,* and certain deficiencies in glycolytic enzymes. (5) Hereditary hemolytic disorders due to hemoglobinopathies mainly affect persons of African, Mediterranean, or Asian descent; the most prevalent of these disorders is *sickle cell anemia,* followed by *hemoglobin C disease,* double heterozygosity for hemoglobins S and C, *hemoglobin E disease,* and a host of uncommon disorders characterized by instability of hemoglobin. (6) Toxicologic hemolytic disorders often (but not exclusively) affecting individuals possessing the genetic defect glucose 6-phosphate dehydrogenase (G6PD) deficiency are known collectively as the *Heinz body hemolytic anemias*. In these, hemoglobin is precipitated as inclusion bodies during exposure to any of a number of oxidant agents. (7) Infection of red cells by organisms such as plasmodia rank among the most dangerous and widespread causes of hemolytic anemias. (8) Splenomegaly may be a consequence or a cause of hemolysis. When a consequence, as in HS, splenic enlargement may critically exacerbate the process. When a cause, as in congestive splenomegaly, hemolysis is moderately increased but most of the anemia is the result of splenic pooling. Anemia accompanying splenic enlargement is best designated *splenomegaly syndrome,* for the mystical term *hypersplenism* is fast falling into desuetude.

Figure 16. Mechanically Induced Hemolysis. Microangiopathic Hemolytic Anemias. Thrombotic Thrombocytopenic Purpura.

A multitude of disorders affecting either the microvasculature or ventricular outflow may cause mechanical fragmentation of red cells and intravascular hemolysis. Widespread, diffuse disease of the arteriolar vessels can lead to abrasion and fracture of flowing blood cells, a process often instigating *disseminated intravascular coagulation* (DIC). With DIC, fibrin and fibrin split products are deposited on the arteriolar surfaces, and vascular lumina may become crisscrossed by fibrin strands, disrupting the pattern of laminar flow. Continued hydraulic hammering creates several characteristic cellular deformities. When individual red cells become draped over fibrin strands, the contents of the suspended cell slump to one side or the other of the transverse "clotheslines." If arteriolar flow is sufficiently forceful, the cell is cleaved at the line of suspension, thereby becoming 2 unequal half-spheroids or *schistocytes*, which on resealing resume circulating. The larger of the cell products are shaped like helmets or bibs. The smaller cell fragments are usually triangular or kite-shaped. The admixture in the blood of numerous *helmet cells* and *fragmented forms* is pathognomonic of *microangiopathic hemolytic anemia*. A most graphic example of intravascular hemolysis induced by mechanical injury is that seen in patients with aortic valve prostheses (**Figure 16-1**, ×1,260), particularly when the prosthesis has torn partly from its aortic moorings, fomenting regurgitant jets and turbulent flow with each heaving heartbeat. Here, the morphologic picture resembles an archaeological harvest. A few cells vaguely resemble military helmets, but the predominant finding is of numerous contracted and pale fragments and shards of every conceivable shape. Many cells are small, dark, scalloped, and vaguely triangular. Some that appear to have been bitten, torn, or pinched in 2 or 3 places resemble acanthocytes. A similar, but less bizarre, collection of red cell deformities is seen uncommonly in patients with incompetent mitral valve prostheses, and mild versions of this "Waring blender syndrome" occur occasionally in physically active patients with calcific aortic stenosis. An acute, self-limited form of intravascular lysis of mechanical origin sometimes arises in young, vigorous persons whose athletic proclivities inspire exceptionally sustained hematologic trauma—so-called *march hemoglobinuria*. In the case of heavy-footed runners stomping for long distances on a hard surface, the specific locale of damage is to blood cells as they pass through vessels in the soles of the feet. Similar violence is done to red cells during other percussive practices such as karate and Conga drumming.

Rheological stress imposed in the microvasculature by *malignant hypertension*, particularly in high-flow organs such as kidneys, may cause extensive damage to red cell membranes, with hemoglobinemia and hemosiderinuria reaching a diurnal maximum in the active, waking hours. As shown in **Figure 16-2** (×800), red cells subjected constantly to harsh impact as they scrape through rigid arterioles at high pressure become fragmented and progressively depleted in membrane. The numerous dark spiny spheroids appear incapable of sustaining many more bumps and concussions without bursting. Note the presence of several smoothly crenulated burr cells, markers of coexistent uremia.

DIC, a human version of the generalized Shwartzman reaction of rabbits, is most commonly encountered in patients suffering from *gram-negative sepsis*. The causes of random, disseminated deposition of fibrin products are legion. Potential precipitators of DIC range from the mundane to the exotic and include such diverse entities as disseminated carcinoma, acute promyelocytic leukemia, preeclampsia, burns, anaphy-laxis, heat stroke, snake (viper) bites, bee stings, acute and chronic glomerulonephritis, renal cortical necrosis, the hemolytic uremic syndrome, favism (in G6PD-deficient Caucasians), botanical poisoning, and photon-mediated lysis. Rarely, DIC may be precipitated by disseminated infection with gram-positive organisms, particularly in patients who were previously splenectomized or whose immune responses were suppressed. Other causative infectious agents are rickettsias, certain viruses, and *Plasmodium falciparum*. All of these are capable of activating a final common pathogenetic pathway marked by the morphologic features shown in **Figure 16-3** (×800). This smear, from a woman in shock from gram-negative sepsis, displays the telltale helmet forms and their companion cell fragments. In addition to helmet cells, there are numerous characteristic burr cells, indicative of the patient's complicating uremia. Note the absence of platelets in this view (denoting thrombocytopenia) and the vacuolated wreckage of a granulocyte, which has detonated most of its granules.

An uncommon, often explosive, and frequently lethal disorder that is a deadly mimic of DIC is *thrombotic thrombocytopenic purpura* (TTP), or Moschcowitz's syndrome. The cardinal features of this frightening disorder of young adults are microangiopathic hemolytic anemia, thrombocytopenic purpura, fluctuating central nervous system crises, fever, and renal failure. TTP appears to be initiated by immunologic damage to endothelium, with release of secretory products that clump platelets and spawn soft platelet-fibrin emboli that lodge in brain, kidneys, and marrow. As exemplified in **Figure 16-4** (×1,260), TTP generates both helmet forms and spherocytes. Because anemia is often severe, large numbers of polychromatophilic and nucleated red cells appear; the latter are partly explained by myelopathic lesions in the marrow. Note the absence of platelets. The combination of helmet cells, nucleated red cells, numerous polychromatophils, and severe thrombocytopenia is strongly suggestive of TTP. As this patient had a hematocrit of only 12 volumes percent, some red cells display the artifactually refractile appearance typical of smears made from thin, watery blood.

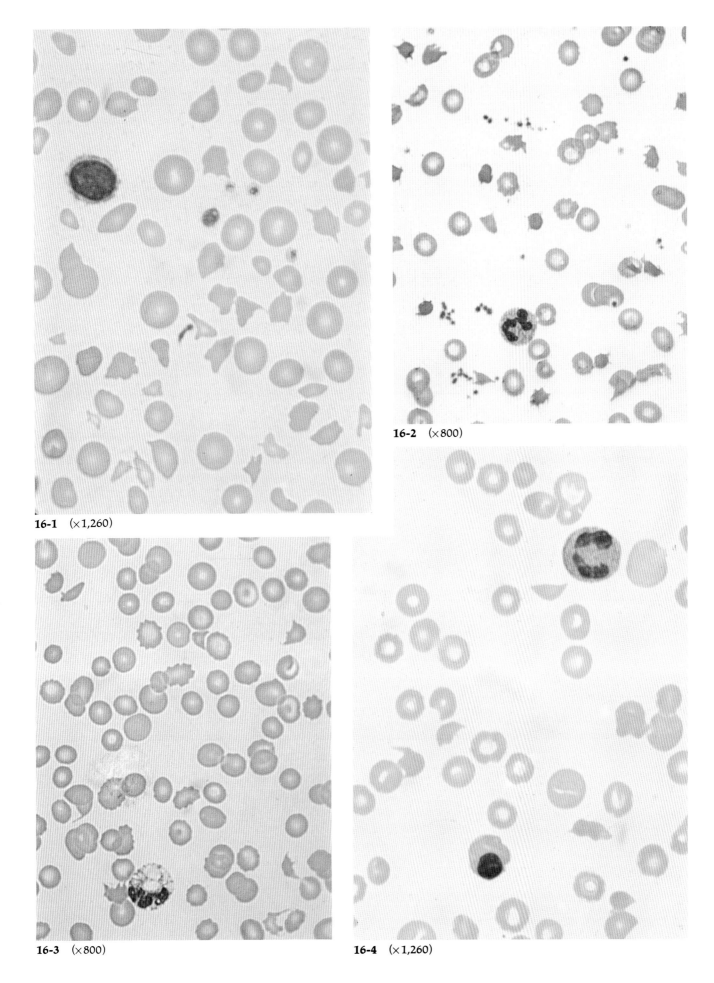

16-1 (×1,260)

16-2 (×800)

16-3 (×800)

16-4 (×1,260)

Figure 17. Immunohemolytic Anemias

Immunohemolytic anemias are caused by attachment of antibodies to red cell surfaces. Subsequent events are determined by the class of antibody and the density and distribution of surface antigens. Most acquired immunohemolytic anemias occur through an immunologic mistake, which somehow engenders antibodies that react nonspecifically with nearly all human red cells, including those of the patient—so-called autoantibodies. In many instances this lapse in toleration is associated with lymphoproliferative disorders, global autoimmune problems such as systemic lupus erythematosus, or a confused immune response to haptenic drugs. Antibodies of the IgM class are most active in the cold, and cell destruction is caused by agglutination or activation of serum complement. Antibodies of the IgG class (Rh antibodies are the prototype) are most reactive at body temperature, and hemolysis is the indirect result of binding of cell-attached IgG molecules by macrophages residing in sinuses of the spleen and liver. Macrophages are equipped with receptors that bind avidly to the protruding Fc (rear) ends of antibodies attached head-down to red cell surfaces. Fc receptor-mediated binding causes red cell membranes to fuse to macrophage surfaces; their membranes are softened and depleted of area by probing microvilli that reach out from the aroused macrophage. Many trapped red cells are either swallowed outright or are nibbled to death piecemeal; others are bound for a time and lose portions of their surface but are then released back and circulate briefly as spherocytes.

The diagnostic cachet of immunohemolytic anemias is the positive *direct Coombs test* (direct antiglobulin test, or DAT). This is an immunologic trick in which heterologous antibodies to human immunoglobulins or to complement components (namely degradation products of C3) are used to bridge together cells coated with proteins having too small a reach to agglutinate cells directly, as do cell-spanning IgM antibodies.

In severe immunohemolytic anemia, the red cell population is a mixture of spherocytes and polychromatophils. **Figures 17-1** ($\times$800) and **17-3** ($\times$2,000) display this extreme dimorphism, showing roughly equal numbers of microspherocytes only 4 to 5 μm across and pale, faintly polychromatophilic macrocytes of more than twice that width. When this cell pattern accompanies an acute hemolytic process, the diagnosis of immunohemolytic anemia can be presumed, subject to confirmation by the Coombs test. The only other hemolytic process associated with such large numbers of smooth spherocytes is hereditary spherocytosis, a disorder usually differentiable by past history and family history. That the large, pale cells of **Figures 17-1** and **17-3** are polychromatophils still possessing stainable ribosomes is substantiated in **Figure 17-2** ($\times$1,260). This figure shows a suspension of patient red cells that were stained by incubating the blood for 10 minutes with an equal volume of an isotonic solution containing 0.5 g/dl of new methylene blue. There are 2 distinct populations of cells. About half are large cells having dark blue inclusions. The remainder are smaller, mostly spheroidal cells that are stained green but do not contain inclusions. The macrocytes with inclusions are reticulocytes and their enumeration yields the reticulocyte count. This approximates the proportion of cells that are polychromatophilic, but some immature red cells that are lightly polychromatophilic on Wright-Giemsa staining do not form reticular clumps on staining with new methylene blue. In busy laboratories, it is acceptable to enumerate reticulocytes by examining suspensions of supravitally stained cells. Quick scanning of stained preparations provides a sufficient indication of the presence or absence of reticulocytes and of any significant increase in their number. Note the hypersegmentation of both neutrophil nuclei in **Figure 17-1**. Hypersegmentation is common in severe hemolytic anemia and reflects a complicating megaloblastic arrest that usually responds to folate.

Blood from a patient who had developed mild hemolytic anemia and a positive anti-C3 Coombs test during convalescence from mycoplasma pneumonia showed prominent agglutination, as pictured in **Figure 17-4** ($\times$1,260). That agglutination occurred ex vivo at ambient temperature and not in vivo at central body temperature was indicated by absence of clumping when blood smears were prepared using equipment prewarmed to 38°C. About 95% of *cold agglutinins* are specific for the I antigen, but some react only with persisting fetal i antigen or with I antigens in combination with other blood group determinants. Despite high titers of these polyclonal IgM kappa antibodies, hemolysis is restrained by the fact that the complement sequence is seldom consummated. Cell destruction is delimited by proteolytic inactivation of cell-bound C3b to the inert but sticky product, C3d, which blocks further binding of the agglutinin. Note that unagglutinated red cells possess normal central pallor, whereas clumped cells appear darkly spheroidal; this appearance is spurious, for after suspensions are warmed the detached red cells are neither spherical nor osmotically fragile. Cold agglutinins produce factitious lowering of the red cell count and marked elevation of the MCV as measured by automated counters. Red cell counts are lowered because doublets and triplets are machine-counted as single cells, and very large clumps are often excluded entirely. Hence, MCV is overestimated and MCHC is underestimated. An anomalously low MCHC should always alert the laboratory staff to search the smear for agglutination.

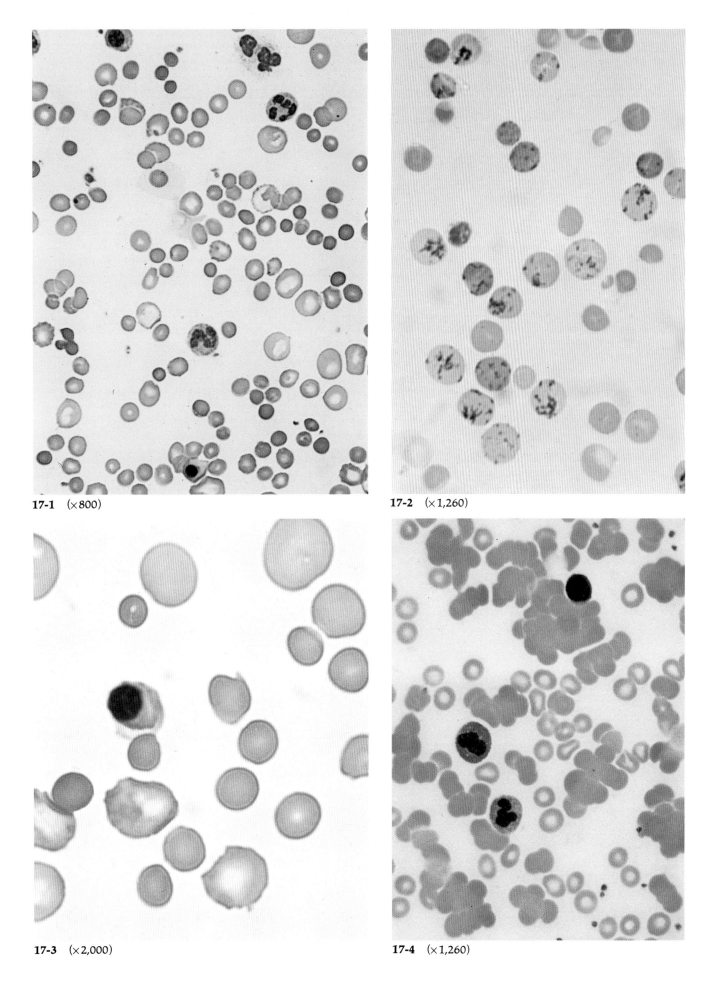

17-1 （×800）

17-2 （×1,260）

17-3 （×2,000）

17-4 （×1,260）

Figure 18. Hereditary Spherocytosis

Hereditary spherocytosis is the most prevalent hemolytic disorder among persons of northern European descent. HS is usually transmitted by a single autosomal dominant gene, but in 25% of cases the disease arises through mutation. In a minority of families, transmission occurs via recessive inheritance, and homozygotes may have transfusion-dependent hemolytic anemia. The molecular defects responsible for HS have not been elucidated fully, but there is ample evidence that HS cells are born with an intrinsic deficit of spectrin and possibly other components of the cytoskeleton. The resultant reduction in surface area imparts a slight native spheroidicity; like fat people, these fat red cells bend with difficulty. When fully expressed, HS is a serious disease causing severe anemia, jaundice, and pigment stones. Severely manifested disease is usually diagnosed in early life, and the hemolytic process can be halted by splenectomy. It is the mild or moderate variants, which constitute over half of the cases of HS, that are most often overlooked, for in the absence of frank anemia, a hematologic examination by use of an automatic particle counter alone usually will miss the diagnosis. Diagnosis depends on recognition of 3 subtle cytologic signs: (1) red cells are increased in thickness and decreased in diameter; (2) the cells show very little central pallor; and (3) the MCHC is higher than normal, usually between 36 and 40 g/dl. All of these features are apparent on a blood smear, where the predominance of small, spheroidal, look-alike cells should catch the eye.

Blood from a patient with moderately severe HS (**Figure 18-1**, ×2,000) is remarkable for the large proportion of spherocytes. This monotony of spherical forms is relieved only by a subpopulation of large, bluish polychromatophils. Spherocytes and their shrunken derivatives, microspherocytes, are unusually susceptible to hypotonic lysis in vitro (i.e., they show increased *osmotic fragility*). In vivo, they had been conditioned by repetitious passage through the cordal compartment of the splenic red pulp, in which crowded crypts they were subjected to stepwise depletion of membrane lipid; this rendered them progressively more osmotically fragile and more vulnerable to eventual retention and cell death in the spleen. Splenic conditioning can be mimicked in vitro by the *incubation fragility test,* in which sterile and static incubation of blood for 24 hours elicits an exaggerated increase in osmotic fragility of HS cells. HS is unique in that the anemia invariably is abolished by an uncomplicated splenectomy. It should be noted that, while splenectomy entirely corrects the anemia in HS and halts hazardous accumulations of bile pigments and of pigment stones in the gallbladder, spheroidicity of the red cells persists as a harmless residuum.

Figure 18-2 is a high-power view (×2,000) of blood from another unsplenectomized patient with HS. This patient was minimally affected: his anemia was mild (hemoglobin concentration varying between 12 and 14 g/dl), and his spells of painless jaundice were few and fleeting. Nevertheless, he is in lifelong peril of experiencing aplastic crises or problems caused by bilirubin gallstones. All of the red cells in this view are to some degree spheroidal. Most lack central pallor and, where some pallor is visible, it is miniscule. Even the best smears of normal blood contain some fields, usually near the outer margins, in which red cells simulate spherocytes. Such facsimiles can be distinguished from true spherocytes because they are broad, pale, and often possess cornered margins.

The monotonous, regimental look of HS red cells is quite apparent under low power (**Figure 18-3**, ×800). All of the red cells are overtly undersized when matched against the nucleus of the normal small lymphocyte at the top of the field, and virtually all are either spheroidal or smoothly spherical. Following a beneficial splenectomy, this patient's red cells underwent characteristic changes (**Figure 18-4**, ×800). Polychromatophils have disappeared, the cells have a more homogeneous red cell volume distribution width (RDW), and 10 to 20% of the cells have acquired spicules. This spiny transformation, reminiscent of acanthocytosis or spur cell anemia, affects a small percentage of red cells postsplenectomy in otherwise normal individuals. In HS after splenectomy, spiculated cells are much more numerous. Surprisingly, despite their deformity, there is no appreciable impairment in survival of these spiculated cells, either in the patient or following transfusion into normal spleenless recipients. Their pathogenesis is explained by the fact that after splenectomy red cells acquire an increase in membrane surface proportional to their increase in lipids, particularly in cholesterol. The cytoskeleton of HS cells is unalterably diminished, however, thus limiting the potential surface area. The surplus of lipids and redundancy of surface area cause the membrane to form prickly protuberances.

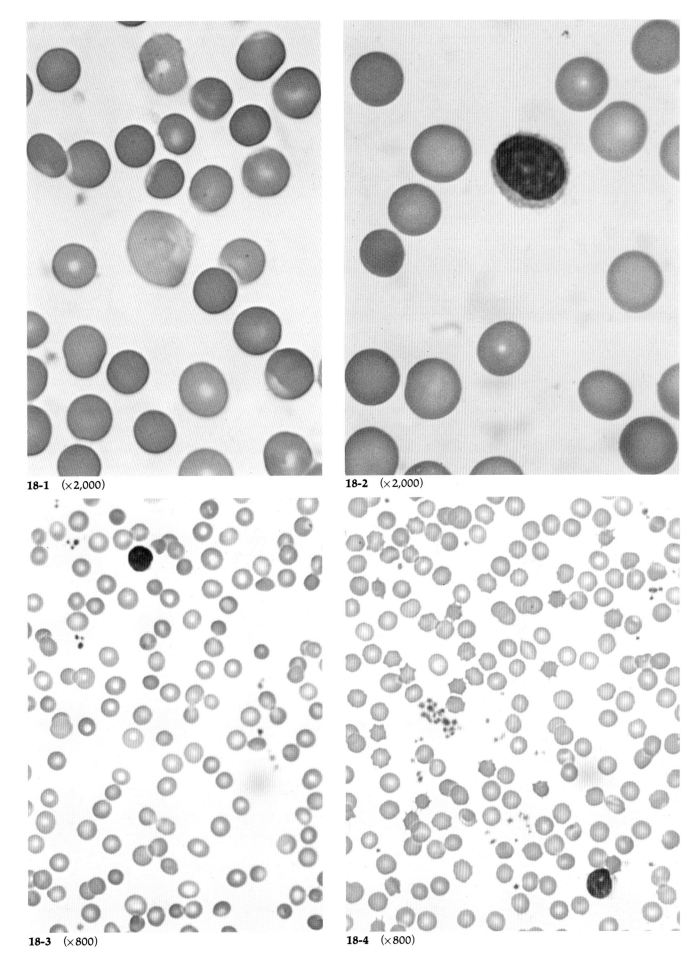

18-1 (×2,000)

18-2 (×2,000)

18-3 (×800)

18-4 (×800)

Figure 19. Hereditary Elliptocytosis. Hereditary Pyropoikilocytosis. Stomatocytosis. Target Cells.

Hereditary elliptocytosis (HE), which is inherited through an autosomal dominant gene, weakens the cytoskeletal structure of red cells, causing them to assume an ellipsoidal shape when they enter the circulation. The lateral skeletal instability and defective shape recovery responsible for red cell elongation are usually caused by a genetic defect in spectrin dimer self-association. Normally the noodle-shaped spectrin molecules are assembled in a stable tetrameric conformation. In the most common HE variants, up to one-third of spectrin exists as dismembered dimers, usually because genetic truncation of spectrin α chains interrupts cytoskeletal lattice formation. Ellipsoidal deformities may occur in uremia, megaloblastic anemia, iron deficiency anemia, thalassemia, and sickle cell anemia, but in none of these disorders are there nearly as many cells affected. Their smaller size and sausage shape clearly differentiate HE cells from the macro-ovalocytes of megaloblastic anemia.

Typical HE cells resemble blunt-ended canoes with sides that are nearly parallel (**Figure 19-1**, ×1,260). The majority of this patient's red cells are ellipsoidal, and at least 25% have a length : width ratio in excess of 2 : 1. Note that the more elongated cells simulate biconcave dumbbells, the hemoglobin being distributed at opposite ends. A mild increase in red cell destruction affects more than half of HE patients, but only about 10% of all patients with HE have frank hemolytic anemia. In these, the usual features of congenital hemolysis are evident: increased reticulocyte levels, erythroid hyperplasia of the marrow, diminished or absent serum haptoglobin, mild intermittent jaundice, and faceted pigment gallstones. In the 1 in 10 patients who have both increased hemolysis and anemia, *microelliptocytes* may be present, as may comma-shaped and teardrop forms. Bizarre budding deformities contribute to the markedly anisocytotic picture. Paradoxically, those HE individuals with the severest hemolysis have so many spherocytes and poikilocytes that there are fewer classic elliptocytic cells. In patients with appreciable hemolytic anemia, the indicated therapy is splenectomy. Uncomplicated splenectomy may not entirely arrest the hemolytic process, but hemolysis is diminished and anemia is either cured or ameliorated, albeit elliptocytosis persists.

Hereditary pyropoikilocytosis (HPP) is a severe congenital hemolytic disorder distinct from but closely related to HE. Most infants with HPP are doubly heterozygous for α chain spectrin defects, and most of their spectrin is in the unstable dimer form. Consequently, aggregates of free spectrin dimers wrapped in membrane are shed from the cells, which become extremely microcytic, many showing characteristic budding or retort-shaped deformities (**Figure 19-2**, ×1,260). Heating HPP red cells briefly at 45 to 46°C exaggerates *budding deformities* and causes the cells to fragment into miniature spherules. Nearly identical budding and fragmentation of red cells into microspherules is seen in patients with widespread *third-degree burns*. Presumably the microspherocytic hemolytic anemia of burn patients represents an analogous destabilization of spectrin taking place at destructively high temperatures. In HPP, virtually every cell is misshapen in some way, but *microspherocytes*, wizened *pyknocytes*, fragments, and elliptocytes predominate. In many cases, as intimated here, the mutilated pyknocytes of HPP are replaced during the first year by the elliptocytes of common HE, with abatement or moderation of hemolysis.

Red cells of a child with congenital hemolytic anemia and *hereditary stomatocytosis* are portrayed in **Figure 19-3** (×1,260). The patient had improved partially after splenectomy, which procedure accounts for the orthochromatic erythroblast and the increase in red cell diameter. Half of the red cells have a linear slot-shaped central area of pallor that confers a mouth-like appearance. Most cells appear to have been folded along the long axis of the stoma, but some appear twice-folded and resemble sleighbells. In suspension, stomatocytes are seen as bowl-shaped, uniconcave, or pocket-shaped cells. Stomatocytosis with mild hemolytic anemia is an unexplained feature of the rare individuals whose red cells lack all Rh antigen determinants (i.e., who are "Rh-null"). Stomatocytosis reflects a membrane disturbance in cation transport and volume control, resulting in accumulation of sodium and over-hydration. These red cells are edematous—hence the growing popularity of the term *hereditary hydrocytosis*.

Target cells (codocytes, Mexican hat cells) are cells of broad diameter and diminished thickness which, in suspension, often appear like flared cups, bowls, or bells but which, on dried smears, have an artifactual bull's-eye appearance. Targeting is most uniform and striking in hemoglobin C disease and in intrahepatic or extrahepatic obstructive jaundice. **Figure 19-4** (×1,260) portrays the blood smear of a patient with pronounced jaundice caused by alcoholic cirrhosis with cholangiolitic obstruction. About half the red cells appear targeted. During biliary obstruction, red cell membranes become overloaded with free (unesterified) cholesterol and sustain a proportional increase in surface area. This spreading of surface does not alter cell volume or suppleness, and, within limits, membrane redundancy does not adversely affect cell survival. Targeting is a harmless artifact of rapid drying, caused by puddling of hemoglobin near the center of excessively broad and thin cells.

The very uniform targeting seen in hemoglobin C disease reflects the same principle, but centroidal puddles form during drying because of the diminished solubility of hemoglobin rather than because of a greater distance to the rim. Targeting can be seen in lesser degree in hemoglobin C trait, in normal individuals postsplenectomy, and in rare individuals having a familial deficiency of lecithin-cholesterol acyltransferase (LCAT). In thalassemic disorders, target cells are plentiful but are intermingled with other aberrant cells.

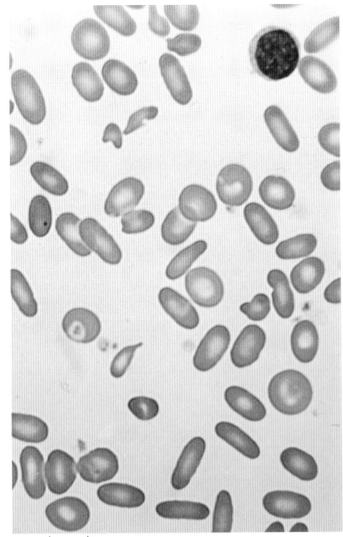

19-1 (×1,260)

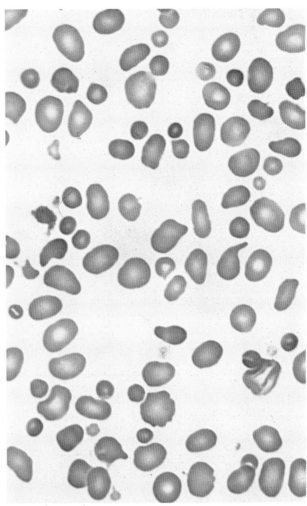

19-2 (×1,260)

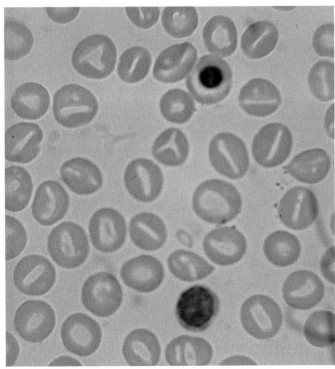

19-3 (×1,260)

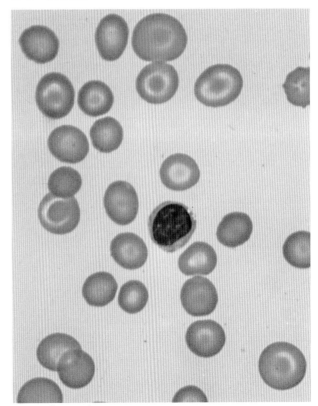

19-4 (×1,260)

Figure 20. Acanthocytes. Spur Cells. Burr Cells.

Acanthocytes are darkly contracted red cells having numerous thorny spicules. These prickly spheroids are a prominent morphologic feature of 2 very different disorders affecting lipid metabolism, *abetalipoproteinemia* and *spur cell anemia*. However dissimilar their pathogenesis and clinical contexts, the acanthocytes found in hereditary abetalipoproteinemia (**Figure 20-1**, ×2,000) are nearly indistinguishable from those of patients with alcoholic cirrhosis and spur cell anemia (**Figure 20-2**, ×2,000).

Abetalipoproteinemia is a rare inborn derangement of lipid metabolism arising from an inability of jejunal mucosa cells to synthesize and assemble the lipid transport protein, apolipoprotein B. This leads to severe reductions in the levels of all major plasma lipids, with a disproportionate diminution in lecithin in exchange for the more rigid lipid, sphingomyelin. The resultant imbalance in membrane lipids causes immature red cells to wrinkle, pucker, stiffen, and spiculate at the moment of their entry into circulation. Despite their lumpy, tasseled appearance, the overall membrane viscosity of these wretched-looking red cells is not increased sufficiently to impede transit in the microcirculation, and hemolysis is mild.

Some patients with advanced hepatocellular disease, usually *alcoholic cirrhosis,* acquire a severe, progressive hemolytic anemia associated with splenomegaly and acanthocytosis. In spur cell anemia an abnormal high-density lipoprotein accumulates that causes excessive unloading of free (unesterified) cholesterol onto red cell membranes. Mild increases in cholesterol and hence surface area cause red cells to spread out harmlessly and to appear flattened and even targeted on smears (see **Figure 19-4**). In cirrhotic patients (and in infants with *neonatal hepatitis*), cholesterol overloading can be extreme; redundancy of the lipid bilayer may exceed the physical limits of the cytoskeletal framework, causing the cell surface to buckle and extend cholesterol-rich protrusions. These stiff spicules are rudely snapped off during repetitious passage through the spleen, transforming the cell to a prickly sphere. Morphologic testimony to the sequence of events described is a mixture of spiculated spherocytes, flat broad cells with wavy or crenulated margins, and smooth bland polychromatophils (**Figure 20-2**).

A rare form of acanthocytosis, unaccompanied by aberrations of membrane lipids or permeability, affects red cells lacking the Kell blood group antigen, K_x. In males with the X-linked phenotype designated McLeod, K_x is absent from red cell membranes, many or most red cells appear acanthocytic, and there may be mild compensated hemolysis. Males whose red cells lack K_x antigen have *chronic granulomatous disease* (CGD), but not all cases of CGD are associated with deficiency of K_x. Mothers of boys having both CGD and McLeod phenotype have a mixture of normal and acanthocytic red cells, as predicted by *Lyon's law.*

Figure 20-3 (×2,000) depicts the conformational changes seen in many or most red cells in patients with uremia. The pathogenesis of this unique shape change is unknown. It may ensue with very slight degrees of azotemia and is a universal feature of uremia, irrespective of etiology or the degree of anemia, if any. Two incompletely linked morphologic abnormalities accompany uremia. Many red cells (usually one third or more) possess a dozen or so even-sized, regularly spaced, smoothly rounded crenulations. The usual term for these serrated cells is *burr cells.* A less apt expression is *echinocyte,* meaning "sea urchin cell" or "urchinoid cell." Ellipsoidal cells are almost as numerous as burr cells, and cells that are both ellipsoidal and serrated often simulate oak leaves. Burr cells are a benign and potentially reversible feature of renal failure. They diminish rapidly during efficacious dialysis and vanish entirely following successful renal transplantation.

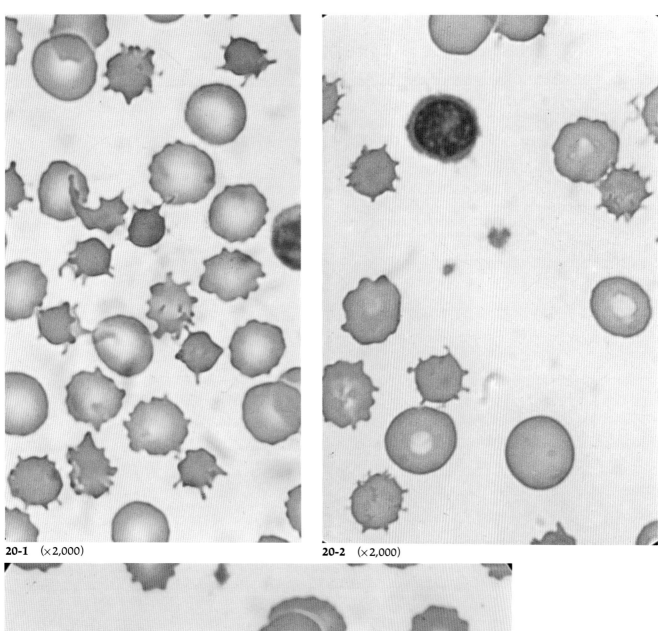

20-1 (×2,000)

20-2 (×2,000)

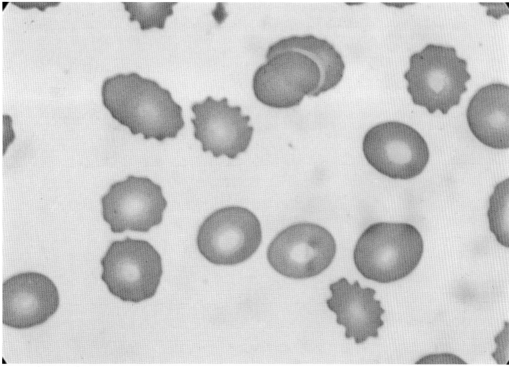

20-3 (×2,000)

Figure 21. Sickle Cell Anemia. Sickle–β Thalassemia.

Inspection of **Figure 21-1** ($\times 800$) permits an unequivocal diagnosis of *sickle cell anemia* (SCA, homozygous hemoglobin S disease, or hemoglobin SS disease). This blood smear is from a young man with anemia and "painful crises" beginning in infancy. The spells of musculoskeletal pain attest to vaso-occlusions by small plugs of entangled, sickled red cells. When deoxygenated at body temperature, SCA red cells soon simulate holly leaves or thin crescents, and then become filamentous and spiculated. These shape changes, particularly if intensified through chemical deoxygenation by sodium metabisulfite (the Daland-Castle test), provide a dependable means for diagnosing sickle cell anemia when used in conjunction with hemoglobin electrophoresis. Arteriolar occlusions by impacted and unyielding aggregates of sickled red cells cause episodes of ischemic pain resembling the "bends" (decompression sickness). These small occlusions in time engender larger blockages and tissue necrosis. Necrotic lesions develop in roughly the following order: the bones show patchy aseptic necrosis and, occasionally, septic necrosis; the spleen is invariably obliterated; the liver sustains multiple red infarcts, often creating hepatic crises; the renal medulla is damaged, and necrotic cavitation of the renal calyces may ensue; and the course is punctuated by bouts of pneumonia. Ultimately the steady march of pulmonary hypertension, cor pulmonale, and progressive right ventricular failure, compounded by recurring bronchopneumonia, ordain a premature demise.

Individuals inheriting a gene for hemoglobin S from 1 parent and a gene for hemoglobin A from the other have *sickle cell trait*. In them, none of the dire pathological events cited above occurs, except for uncommon instances of delimited renal medullary infarction with hematuria. The health and life expectancy in persons with sickle cell trait, which affects 7 to 8% of black Americans, is normal, and sickle-shaped cells do not appear in capillary or arterial blood.

Figure 21-1 displays a dozen or so eye-catching, sharply crescentic forms known as *irreversibly sickled cells* (ISCs), the logos of sickle cell anemia. Their dark ropey appearance is acquired during sustained hypoxia in the microcirculation, as polymerized deoxyhemoglobin S is assembled into macroscopic fibrils long enough to extend the cell. Polymerization of hemoglobin S increases the leak rate of SCA cells for cations and thereby immortalizes their angular deformity through desiccation. Other deformities characteristic of sickling include splinter shapes, pointed ellipsoids, and long, dark, twisted cells resembling croissants. Amid the farrago of elongated forms are several target cells and numerous broad red cells with increased areas of central pallor. The appearance of hypochromia is illusory. These pale, flat cells reflect the combined effects of increased cell diameter (due to "absence" of the spleen) and diminished solubility of hemoglobin S. The 2 orthochromatic erythroblasts with pyknotic nuclei and the cell with Pappenheimer bodies (top center) are also consequences of asplenia. White counts are persistently elevated in uninfected adults with sickle cell anemia, characteristically being between 15,000 and 25,000 white cells per µl. Modest eosinophilia is common.

In the United States, the incidence of sickle cell anemia at birth is estimated at roughly 1,600 per million black Americans; because of diminished life expectancy, the prevalence is about 600 to 800 per million. Some patients have mild, symptomless courses, despite inheritance of 2 genes for hemoglobin S. The severity of SCA is determined by the level and distribution among red cells of fetal hemoglobin. Among the "fortunate" minority having even as little as 4 to 5% hemoglobin F, the severity of the disease may be moderated, and in those with hemoglobin F levels of 10 to 20%, SCA may be nearly silent. Full, unqualified protection by hemoglobin F against harm from sickle cell anemia is provided only to those rare individuals whose S-hemoglobinopathy is offset by inheritance of an allelic gene for hereditary persistence of fetal hemoglobin (HPFH). **Figure 21-2** ($\times 800$) depicts the blood of a patient homozygous for hemoglobin S with mild anemia, infrequent painful crises, and 8% hemoglobin F. There are some elongated cells, but only 1 (bottom left) has a vaguely crescentic shape. Present also are some target cells, several poikilocytes and fragmented forms, and a few squared-off and holly forms presumed to contain short polymers of hemoglobin S. The patient's white cell count was elevated (22,000 per µl); absence of toxic granulation and Döhle bodies suggests that this reflects "autosplenectomy" rather than infection.

The most common cause of sickle cell syndrome in persons of Mediterranean descent is double heterozygosity for hemoglobin S and β thalassemia (*microdrepanocytic* or *sickle–β-thal disease*). Hemolysis may be moderately severe, and patients experience the full gamut of sickling afflictions. In contrast to SCA, splenomegaly is prominent, explaining the comparative paucity of classic ISCs in unsplenectomized patients. As shown in **Figure 21-3** ($\times 800$), the blood smear reveals marked hypochromia, microcytosis, targeting, teardrop deformities, and some darkly flattened or fusiform cells but only occasional ISCs (right center). Most doubly heterozygous patients have sickle-β⁺-thal and the finding on electrophoresis of some hemoglobin A in addition to hemoglobins S and F confirms the diagnosis. Differentiation of SCA from *sickle–β⁰-thal* is harder because only hemoglobins S and F (plus a trace of A_2) are present in both. The issue can be resolved by family studies showing that one parent has sickle cell trait and the other β thalassemia minor.

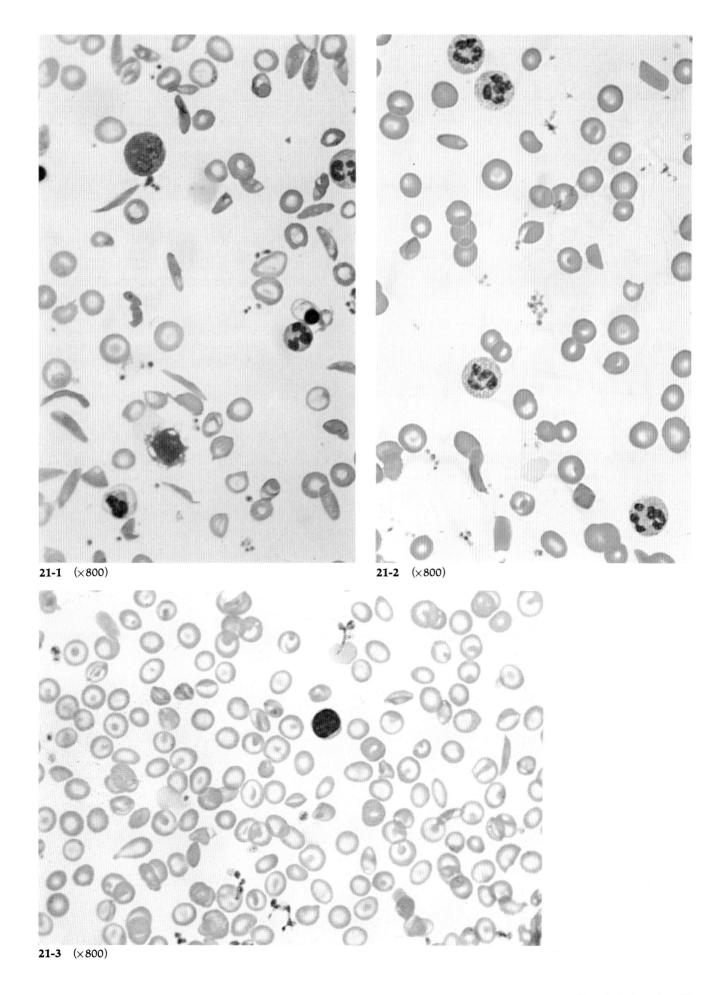

21-1 （×800）

21-2 （×800）

21-3 （×800）

Figure 22. Hemoglobin SC Disease. Hemoglobin C Disease. Hemoglobin C Trait. Hemoglobin E Disease.

Figure 22-1 (×800) portrays the peripheral blood in the doubly heterozygous disorder *hemoglobin SC disease*. Caused by inheritance of a hemoglobin S gene from 1 parent and a hemoglobin C gene from the other, hemoglobin SC disease is not quite as prevalent in the United States as is sickle cell anemia (SCA). In portions of west equatorial Africa, notably Ghana, where genes for hemoglobin C and hemoglobin S are both prevalent, hemoglobin SC disease is at least as common as SCA. The manifestations of hemoglobin SC disease are those of mild or moderate SCA. Painful crises are less frequent and seldom as agonizing: about one-third of SC disease patients never experience musculoskeletal pains and, in another third, commencement of painful crises is delayed until adulthood. Aseptic necrosis of the femoral head and infarctions in renal medulla are about half as common as in sickle cell anemia. Because hemoglobin SC disease generally does not prohibit strenuous use of the arms, the occurrence of aseptic necrosis of the humoral heads is actually more common than in the chronically enervating SCA. In anemic individuals with SC disease, splenomegaly is usually prominent and persists into adulthood in more than half of patients, whereas in SCA patients spleens are so ravaged by major arterial infarctions as to be reduced to sclerotic nubs by late childhood. In SC disease painful splenic infarcts are common, particularly in adults. As in SCA, ischemic damage to the placenta is frequent and predisposes to fetal loss through prematurity, stillbirth, and many other complications of pregnancy. In splenomegalic patients, splenic function is generally enhanced, and the most rigidly deformed red cells are cleared from the bloodstream and collect in splenic sinuses. Hemolytic anemia is moderate and reticulocytosis is restrained. Red cell indices are normal apart from a slight but influential rise in MCHC. As shown in **Figure 22-1**, red cells appear somewhat dense on smear, nearly half are targeted, many look spheroidal, and a few (not shown) may contain hemoglobin crystals. Absent the last, hemoglobin SC disease must be diagnosed by hemoglobin electrophoresis, which reveals about equal amounts of hemoglobin S and the slower-moving hemoglobin C, which comigrates with A_2 and E.

In no other disorder is red cell targeting as startling as in *hemoglobin C disease*. The blood smear (**Figure 22-2**, ×800) shows a major population of bold target forms admixed with smaller numbers of dark spherocytes, many of which appear cracked or nuggety. This pattern is indicative of homozygosity for hemoglobin C, a diagnosis established by finding on electrophoresis that nearly all red cell pigment is hemoglobin C, A being absent. Patients with hemoglobin C disease have mild hemolytic anemia and splenomegaly but are spared the agonies of sickling and the infirmities of thalassemia. Hemolysis of red cells in the spleen is caused by the poor solubility of hemoglobin C; this, in complicity with a unique cation pumping pathway that desiccates the cell, promotes eventual precipitation of the pigment into flat crystals that stack like cards. In contrast to hemoglobin S, hemoglobin C aggregates are formed of oxyhemoglobin; the crystals melt when the cells are deoxygenated, aiding their escape from the clutches of the spleen. Red cells sufficiently stiffened by desiccation when they enter the spleen are subjected to splenic conditioning, with further dehydration and loss of membrane before their release, and eventually repeated conditioning leads to the pyknotic spherocytes seen in **Figure 22-2**. In time, single, block-shaped hexahedral or duodecahedral crystals of hemoglobin may occupy the entire cell. The brick-shaped crystal shown in **Figure 22-3** (×2,000) is pathognomonic of hemoglobin C disease. Suspending red cells of patients with hemoglobin C disease, or even with hemoglobin C trait, in hyperosmolar solutions of sodium citrate or sodium chloride causes polyhedral, birefringent crystals to appear in more than half the red cells, their occurrence under such conditions serving as a diagnostic test.

Hemoglobin C occurs almost solely in blacks, the structural gene mutation of the β chain having originated in northern Ghana and nearby Upper Volta regions. Estimates of the prevalence of hemoglobin C disease depend strongly on the adequacy of population sampling. In the racially mixed population of the Western hemisphere, hemoglobin C is second in prevalence only to hemoglobin S. Among black Americans 2.4% are heterozygous for hemoglobins A and C and 0.02% have homozygous hemoglobin C disease. Hemoglobin C trait is harmless and without hemolysis. This diagnosis is made either by chance or in the course of family studies and should be suspected whenever excessive targeting is found in the absence of hypochromia or spherocytosis. As typified in **Figure 22-4** (×2,000), the blood usually shows 30 to 40% target cells in an otherwise benign-looking smear. Note at the lower left the chance superimposition of 2 platelets over 1 red cell. The halo effect of platelets impressed on red cells may lead one to mistake them for parasites.

Hemoglobin E is the most prevalent hemoglobin variant in subtropical Asia and *hemoglobin E disease* is commonly encountered in Americans of Southeast Asian descent. Hemoglobin E is analogous in pathogenesis to β⁺-thalassemia, but anemia is invariably mild and notable mainly for striking microcytosis and uniform targeting (**Figure 22-5**, ×1,260). The morphology is reminiscent of hemoglobin C disease, but target forms are less bizarre and spherocytes are sparse. These 2 hemoglobins comigrate on cellulose acetate but not in citrate agar.

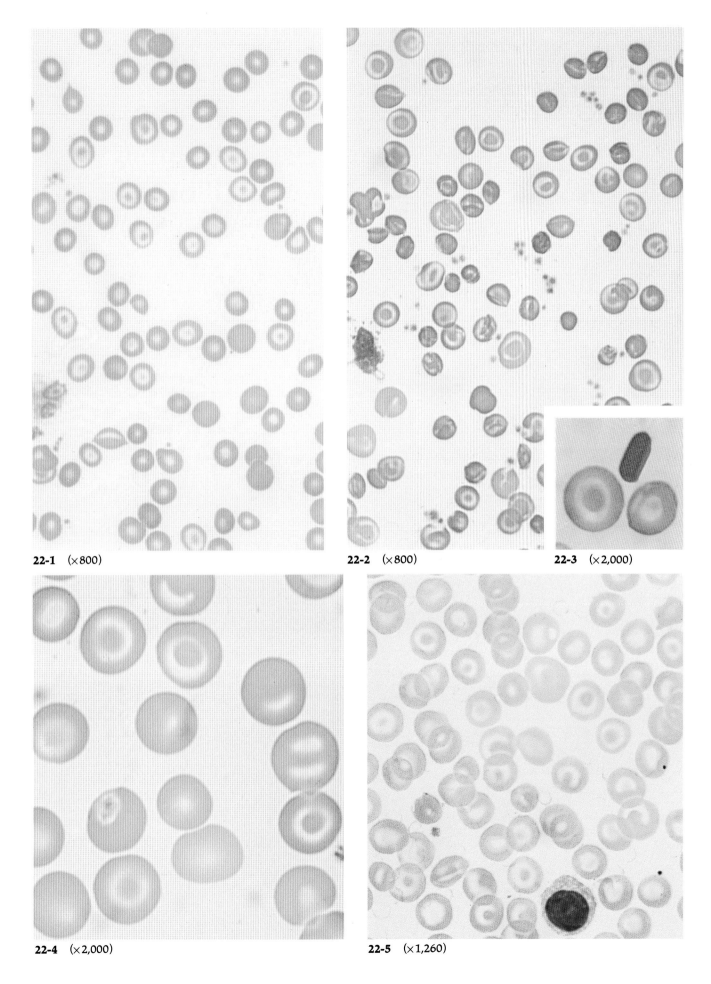

22-1 (×800)

22-2 (×800)

22-3 (×2,000)

22-4 (×2,000)

22-5 (×1,260)

Figure 23. Heinz Bodies. G6PD Deficiency. Favism. Congenital Heinz Body Hemolytic Anemia.

Presence in blood smears of red cells showing 1 or more deep rounded notches is a telltale sign that large inclusion bodies had been bitten out or forcibly pulled off. *Bite-out deformities* bear witness to prior precipitation of either globin chains or hemoglobin. Globin chain deposits and the scars of their removal are found in thalassemias and can be readily identified by the associated thalassemic morphology (see **Figure 13-1**). The finding of bite-out deformities in otherwise normal-looking red cells in the context of acute hemolysis signifies *Heinz body hemolytic anemia* (**Figure 23-1**, ×2,000). **Figure 23-1** shows a red cell with a single bite-out deformity (bottom center), 2 of the cells in **Figure 23-3** (×2,000) have sustained double bites, and 1 red cell at the top right of **Figure 23-4** (×2,000) appears badly chewed up. These 3 fields contain several cells each that appear spheroidal or contracted, but it is the variously bitten cells that betray the pathogenesis of hemolysis.

Heinz bodies are aggregates of hemoglobin precipitated by oxidation. A few of these inclusions within a cell are harmless initially, but within hours they become bonded to the membrane skeleton, reducing cellular resilience. Membrane-bound inclusions soon pout from the cell and then are torn off during the hydraulic battering sustained in the circulation. In the crowded aisles of the spleen, cells containing bags of inclusions are either trapped by their tails, or the tethers snap, releasing wounded but resealed corpuscles bearing mementos of their encounter.

Red cells are designed metabolically to transport oxygen without being burned by it. This is achieved through mechanisms for detoxifying oxygen, which depend ultimately on the rate-limiting enzyme of the hexose monophosphate shunt pathway, G6PD. Entry into red cells of actual or potential oxidant drugs such as sulfonamides, antimalarials, and certain analgesics may short-circuit or overwhelm the antioxidative mechanisms and lead to accumulation of oxidant free radical metabolites of oxygen. If the level of oxidant free radicals is exceptionally high, if the activity of a key defensive enzyme such as G6PD is subnormal, or if hemoglobin is structurally unstable, stepwise oxidations occur, eventuating in precipitation of hemoglobin as Heinz bodies. By the time patients present with hemolytic problems, most badly damaged red cells have been destroyed, and survivors have lost their inclusions through exocytosis. At this juncture the discovery of bite-out deformities, evidence of hemoglobin oxidation to *methemoglobin* and *sulfhemoglobin*, and a history of exposure to potentially oxidant drugs should inspire a diagnosis of *oxidative hemolysis*. The task then is to search for a mechanism predisposing to Heinz body formation, the most common of which is renal failure with impaired excretion of the oxidant. The most prevalent genetic predisposition to oxidative hemolysis is G6PD deficiency, which affects more than 100 million of the world population.

G6PD is encoded by genes on the X chromosome, and thus G6PD deficiency is fully expressed in hemizygous males and homozygous females. The most prevalent G6PD variant, denoted G6PD A-, affects 12% of American black males and is the commonest cause of drug-induced hemolysis among blacks. Among families of Mediterranean descent, the prevalence of G6PD^Med ranges from 3 to 30%. In both of these common forms of G6PD deficiency, the enzyme deficit is harmless unless the individual is exposed to oxidant medications or the enzyme instability is worsened by acute febrile infection or ketoacidosis. Certain variants of G6PD deficiency, such as G6PD^Med (but notably not the A- variant of black individuals) predispose to acute episodes of hemolysis triggered by exposure to the common broad bean *Vicia fava*. Fava beans contain oxidative pyrimidine aglycones that cause hemoglobin aggregation, bite-out deformities, and spherocytosis indistinguishable from those caused by oxidant medication, as illustrated in **Figure 23-4**. *Acute favism* is associated with all the trappings of intravascular hemolysis including hemoglobinemia, hemoglobinuria, and, occasionally, erythrophagocytosis, as featured in **Figure 23-5** (×2,000). Not all G6PD-deficient persons are at risk of suffering acute favism after ingestion of the beans or inhalation of pollen; hemolytic reactions are inconstant, subject to an additional, possibly immunologic, caprice.

Congenital Heinz body hemolytic anemia (CHBHA) is an uncommon disorder caused by inherited aberrations of globin structure that predispose the hemes to oxidation. Hemolysis may be lifelong or may occur only following exposure to oxidant drugs such as sulfonamides. Inclusions of structurally unstable hemoglobins are unusually large and irregular and are most numerous in reticulocytes. Simple screening tests for demonstrating hemoglobin instability include thermal denaturation at 50°C and precipitation in buffered isopropanol.

Oxidative hemolysis is usually suspected from historical circumstance and the finding on blood smears of bite-out deformities. Heinz bodies are not visible on Wright-Giemsa stained smears and may or may not be detectable using supravital dyes. If blood is sampled within the first day or two after ingestion of sufficient oxidant medication, however, numerous characteristic inclusions may be seen following supravital staining of red cells with methyl (or crystal) violet (**Figure 23-2**, ×2,000). Note how the black-stained inclusions tend to adhere to each other and to bulge from the cell surface. Their outward position dooms the cell to deformation and death.

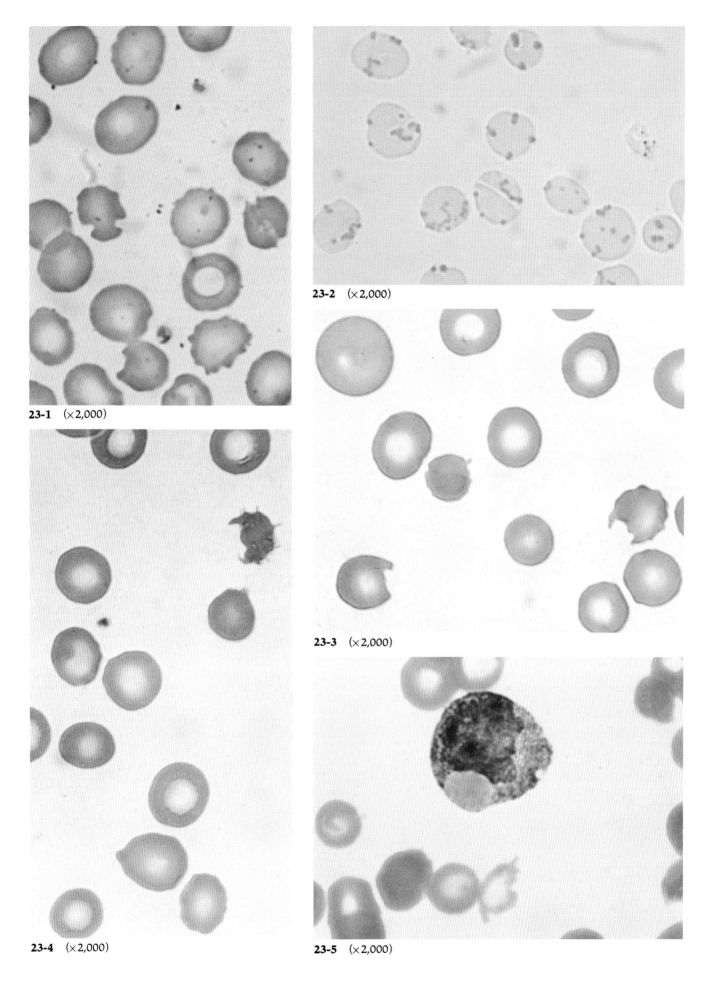

23-1 (×2,000)

23-2 (×2,000)

23-3 (×2,000)

23-4 (×2,000)

23-5 (×2,000)

Figure 24. Malaria. Trypanosomiasis. Babesiosis.

Discovery of exotic nucleated structures within red cells (**Figures 24-1** through **24-4** and **Figures 24-6** and **24-7**) signifies infection by sporozoans. Long serpentine creatures found amid (not within) red cells that look as though they might slither away—and in wet preparations may do so—are either hemoflagellates (**Figure 24-5**) or, if extremely large, nematodes such as the multinucleated microfilariae of filariasis. Malaria, a protozoan infection endemic among nearly half the world's population, is caused by 4 species of the genus *Plasmodium*: *P. vivax*, *P. falciparum*, *P. malariae*, and *P. ovale*. Infective sporozoites enter the bloodstream via the saliva of feeding female anopheles mosquitoes. Organisms also gain entry through blood transfusions. Sporozoites are cleared from the circulation by liver cells, wherein they proliferate through schizogeny. After about 1 week, myriad merozoites are released by the schizonts. These enter red cells through receptor-mediated endocytosis, creating for themselves hospitable vacuoles. Now named *trophozoites*, intraerythrocytic parasites acquire ring shapes and feed on hemoglobin, excreting brownish ferriheme (hematin). The morphology of ring forms and their descendants differs among malarial species: only the 2 most prevalent, *P. vivax* and *P. falciparum*, are described here.

Trophozoites of *P. vivax*, authors of benign tertian malaria, usually occur singly, but sometimes 2 ring forms appear in 1 red cell (**Figure 24-1**, ×2,000). The delicate blue rings are hoop-shaped ellipsoids, 3 to 4 μm across. *P. vivax* preferentially inhabits reticulocytes; thus, host cells are large to begin with and often display polychromatophilia and basophilic stippling. Most rings possess 1 red chromatin dot, which imparts a signet-ring appearance. As trophozoites mature, the red cells double in size, become pale and oblong, and often are freckled by scores of reddish granules (*Schüffner's dots*). Growing trophozoites extend filamentous cytoplasmic processes (pseudopodia), which assume complex, looping configurations, and the ring structure is lost. As the chromatin mass enlarges and undergoes vacuolation, *ameboid trophozoites* eventually attain the size of lymphocyte nuclei. Multiple separated masses of condensed chromatin emerge (*schizogeny*), held together by strands of parasite cytoplasm, and clumps of hematin pile up. **Figures 24-2** and **24-3** (both ×2,000) show *early (presegmenting) schizonts*. Note fading of the dying red cells, the pale blue parasite cytoplasm, the multiple, purple chromatin masses, and clumps of golden hematin *(malarial pigment)*. As the doomed red cells disintegrate, schizonts release their cargo of segments; these *merozoites* are now freed to infect virginal red cells. Separate from the process of *asexual schizogeny*, a few "chosen" parasites undertake *sexual schizogeny* by transforming into large *gametocytes*, each possessing a pale lilac nucleus. The blue cytoplasm of female *macrogametocytes* is more abundant than that of male *microgametocytes*, and nuclear chromatin is more concentrated.

P. falciparum (malignant tertian) malaria is more severe than the others, for many more red cells are initially parasitized. It does not undergo cyclic relapses, and once the erythrocytic cycle of falciparum malaria is over, parasitemia does not recrudesce. In falciparum malaria, late trophozoites and schizonts are rare, whereas all parasite stages coexist in the blood during vivax malaria. Falciparum ring forms are smaller than vivax forms. Multiple infection of red cells is common, marginal (appliqué) forms are numerous, and gametocytes appear shortly after clinical onset. Crescentic or fusiform gametocytes are diagnostic of falciparum malaria. The female macrogametocyte (**Figure 24-4**, ×2,000) is longer and more crescentic than its smaller male counterpart. Its cytoplasm is bluer at the extremities, and the chromatin and yellow pigment are more compact and centralized. Unlike *P. vivax*, *P. falciparum* does not enlarge red cells; indeed, microspherocytes are prevalent. Maurer's dots, which are bolder, darker, and fewer than Schüffner's dots, may appear in the relatively few mature trophozoites visible in falciparum malaria.

Finding the flagellar protozoan responsible for *Gambian trypanosomiasis* (mid-African sleeping sickness) in the blood is the simplest means of diagnosing that dread disorder. A horrid cluster of *Trypanosoma gambiense* is shown in **Figure 24-5** (×2,000). As with malaria, trypanosomal organisms may be so few as to escape detection on routine blood smears. This difficulty can be circumvented by using thick smears prepared on glass slides and clarifying the obscuring layers of red cells by adding water or saponin to the unfixed smear before Wright-Giemsa staining.

Babesiosis (piroplasmosis) is an acute hemolytic disorder of the temperate north caused by several species of small protozoa, the most prevalent of which is *Babesia microti*. *Babesia* are transmitted during blood meals of female hard ticks of the family *Ixodidae* that infest deer or mice. Tickbites inoculate sporozoites into the victim's bloodstream; organisms penetrate red cell membranes via a complement receptor-mediated mechanism, and interiorized trophozoites assume ring shapes very similar to those of *P. falciparum*. Particularly in those patients lacking spleens, babesiosis can cause catastrophic intravascular hemolysis marked by extreme parasitemia, prostration, and frequently death within a week of onset. In individuals with spleens, the disease ranges in intensity from a severe, but usually self-limited, hemolytic anemia to a mild or subclinical febrile illness. Nearly half of the red cells of an asplenic patient with severe babesiosis contain *B. microti* ring forms in **Figures 24-6** and **24-7** (both ×1,500). Note that signet-ring and earring-shaped babesian forms might be mistaken at first for falciparum trophozoites. However, *Babesia* are smaller (diameters, 1.2 to 2.0 μm), hematin pigment is absent even in mature parasites, and there are no schizonts or gametocytes. *Babesia* divide by budding, rather than by schizogeny, each parasite generating a maximum of 4 merozoites. This process propagates a limited assortment of small ring forms. Among these are single rings with single dots, double rings joined by a single chromatin mass, and tetrad forms in which 4 compact masses of purple chromatin are held together by frail strands of blue cytoplasm. Although not numerous, tetrads ("Maltese cross forms") are diagnostic of babesiosis.

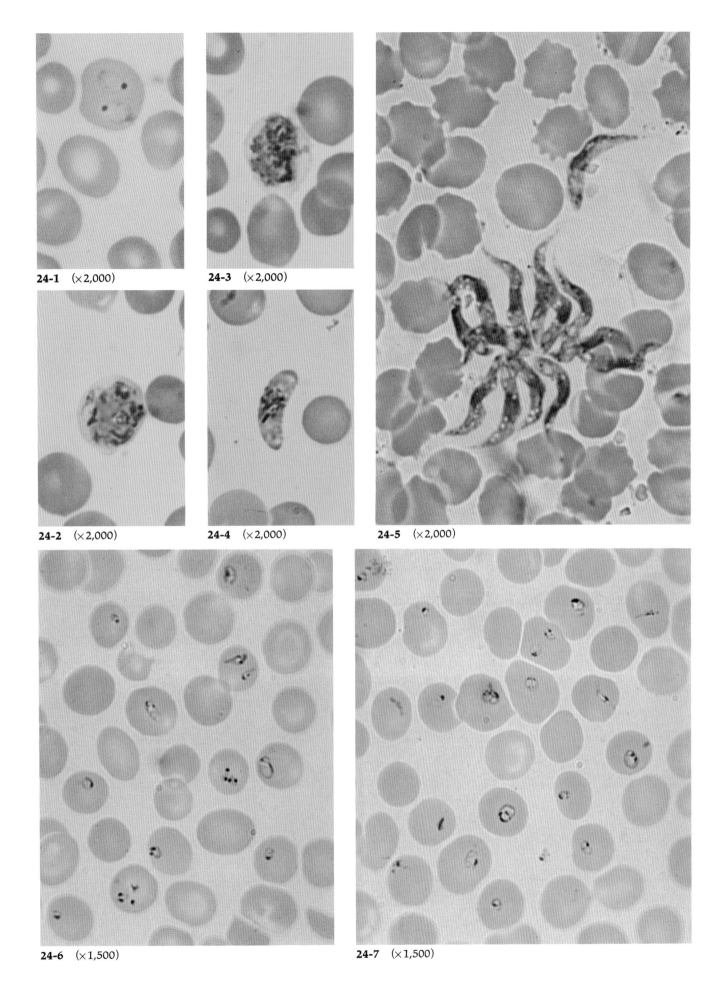

24-1 (×2,000)

24-3 (×2,000)

24-2 (×2,000)

24-4 (×2,000)

24-5 (×2,000)

24-6 (×1,500)

24-7 (×1,500)

Figure 25. Toxoplasmosis. Histoplasmosis. Bartonellosis.

Two ubiquitous microorganisms representing 2 different kingdoms with which humanity is ordinarily at peace are the protozoan *Toxoplasma gondii* (**Figures 25-1** and **25-3**, both ×2,000) and the fungus *Histoplasma capsulatum* (**Figure 25-2**, ×2,000). Both agents are endemic worldwide, kept quiet by the constraints of immunity, but both are capable of decimating the ranks of the immunocompromised. These indolent organisms feast on patients whose cell-mediated immune mechanisms have been depressed by drugs or *human immunodeficiency virus* (HIV) *infection*.

In the immunosuppressed patient, *T. gondii* is an opportunistic pathogen that invades all cells and tissues and inflicts particularly devastating neurologic damage. In patients with *acquired immunodeficiency syndrome* (AIDS), toxoplasmosis causes diffuse necrotizing encephalitis. Diagnosis is often frustrated by the vagaries of serologic tests in AIDS patients and by the extreme difficulty in identifying these obligate intracellular organisms in tissue sections. *T. gondii* can be isolated by inoculating small mammals or by tissue culture, but the most immediate and decisive evidence is obtained by direct examination of infected host cells. **Figure 25-1** is a centrifuged (cytospin) preparation of spinal fluid from a patient with *AIDS encephalopathy*. In the ruins of this squashed macrophage are side-by-side clusters of phagocytized *T. gondii tachyzoites* (trophozoites), with their nuclei characteristically aligned in 2s and 4s, signifying binary divisions. The foursome shown at bottom-center are pathognomonic of toxoplasmosis. The shape of the organism and its characteristic dimensions (about 3 by 6 μm) are more evident in the flattened neutrophils shown in **Figure 25-3**. Note the crescentic and fusiform shapes of the tachyzoites, their deep blue cytoplasm, and the compact central position of their nuclei, some of which are engaged in mitosis. Reactivation of dormant toxoplasmosis in immunosuppressed patients unleashes a pervasive, necrotizing process capable of damaging every organ in the body; for lack of adequate serologic tests in patients progressing rapidly into coma, the finding of phagocytized organisms in spinal fluid or blood can prove crucial to therapy.

Infection by the dimorphic fungus *H. capsulatum* is spread by inhaling dust contaminated with droppings from bats or unpleasant suburban birds such as starlings. Mycelial (mold) forms in soil sprout and release an aerosol of spores that, when ingested by macrophages, transform into thin-walled spherules of yeast. Yeast forms lack a true capsule, ironically, and are nearly invisible in H&E sections. In Wright-Giemsa stained marrow smears, however, macrophages stuffed to the bursting point with scores or hundreds of yeast forms are readily discovered (**Figure 25-2**). Histoplasma yeast forms imprisoned within phagosomal bubbles are quite variable in size (2 to 5 μm across) and shape, and many nuclei resembling larvae or commas and an assortment of single budding forms or hourglass figures may be present. The tiny (2 μm across) amastigotes of the protozoan responsible for *visceral leishmaniasis (kala-azar)*, the trypanosome *Leishmania donovani*, also flourish within the forgiving phagosomes of macrophages. These haloed inclusions known as *Leishman-Donovan bodies* resemble yeast forms at first glance but differ in possessing both a rodlike nucleus and a piece of extranuclear DNA known as a *kinetoplast* or *parabasal body*. These paired purple organelles are pathognomonic structures.

For those who venture into the Andean slopes of Peru, Colombia, or Ecuador at altitudes between 700 and 2,500 m, the sudden onset of hectic fever and prostrating hemolytic anemia should call to mind a diagnosis of *bartonellosis (Car-rión's disease)*. *Bartonella bacilliformis*, a small pleomorphic gram-negative organism, is extremely avid for red cell surfaces. During the acute onslaught, bartonella organisms in multiple shapes swarm over the surfaces of red cells. Spun about by long polar flagellae, the bacilli bore their way into the doomed red cells, converting them to spherocytes in their last moments before "exsanguination." With severe bacteremia, dozens of organisms may feed on each red cell. At the time patients are first seen, blood smears show pronounced spherocytosis, polychromatophilia, and an assortment of dark purple organisms attached to the cell surfaces (**Figure 25-4**, ×2,000). In this figure several red cells are under attack by coccoid and filamentous forms, some of which (midleft) are curved along the outer aspect of the victimized cell. The restricted ecology of bartonellosis is determined by the lifestyle of its diminutive vector—crepuscular female sandflies of the genus *Phlebotomus*. Acute bartonellosis is dangerous if not treated promptly with antibiotics. Survivors are often subjected to a delayed and unsightly dermal eruption known as *verruga peruana*.

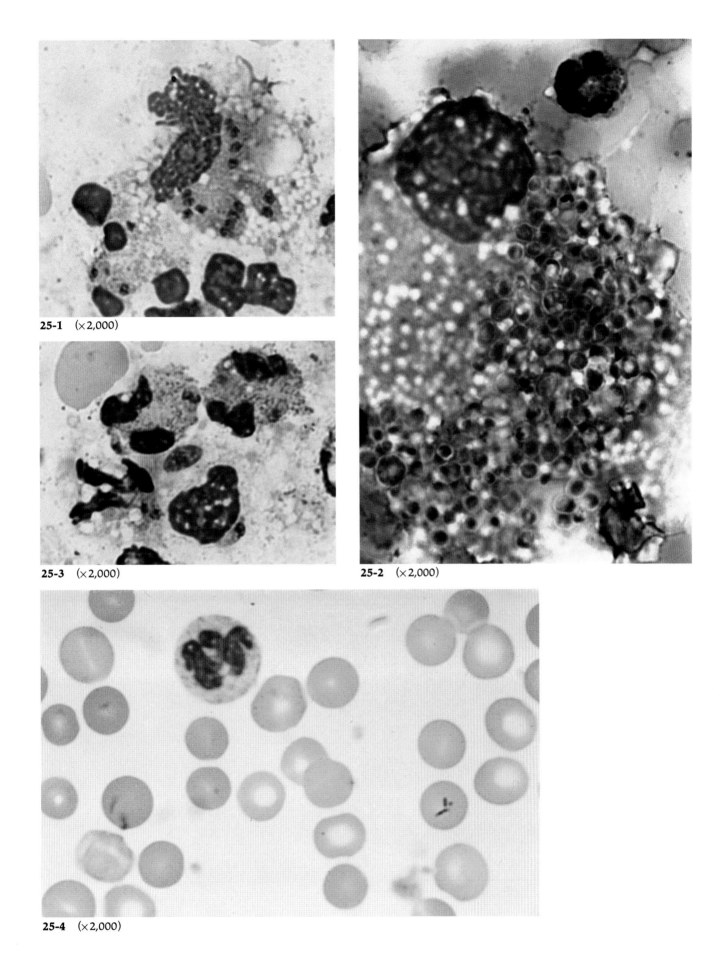

25-1 (×2,000)

25-3 (×2,000)

25-2 (×2,000)

25-4 (×2,000)

Aplastic Anemia and Other Causes of Marrow Failure

Figure 26. Aplastic Anemia

Chronic progressive pancytopenia usually signifies marrow failure—absence or malfunction of hematopoietic stem cells. This morbid process may be caused by simple attrition of marrow parenchyma with replacement by fat (**Figure 26-1**, ×200), physical eviction of marrow stem cells by malignancy or fibrosis, or repopulation of marrow space by clonally transformed dysplastic precursors (*myelodysplasia*).

Aplastic anemia of the classic sort is caused by wasting of all 3 major cell lines—erythroid, myeloid, and megakaryocytic: hence the term *trilineage aplasia*. When the numbers of pluripotential stem cells in marrow drop below about 10% of normal, blood counts decline at rates reflecting the intrinsic lifespans of cells affected. With acute stem cell failure, as may be caused by myelopathic drugs, radiation, or infection, neutrophil and platelet counts are first to fall, leading to secondary infections and thrombocytopenic purpura. More often, the course is one of stalking progression in which anemia is the predominant quantitative feature and the most informative prognostic indicator. In endstage aplasia low-power views of marrow reveal a jellied expanse of adipocytes, with few parenchymal cells visible in H&E–stained biopsy sections (**Figure 26-1**). In assessing marrow cellularity there is no substitute for histologic sections, for the entire geography of the sample can be scanned. Cellularity of this sample is well below 5% (normal range, 40 to 60%), most of the area being occupied by balloonlike adipocytes, which throw into relief vascular structures and stromal scaffolding. Needle biopsy is unsurpassed for quantitating cellularity and is essential to making an unequivocal diagnosis of aplastic anemia. H&E–stained formalin-fixed sections do not lend themselves to making subtle cytologic distinctions, however, because of shrinkage artifacts, their limited red-blue color spectrum, and dissolution of telltale organelles such as the blackish granules of mast cells. The complementary value of a Wright-Giemsa–stained aspirate of the same marrow is illustrated in **Figure 26-3** (×800). Panoptic staining of air-dried smears reveals that most survivors in this ravaged marrow are lymphocytes, accompanied by smaller numbers of plasma cells (lower left) and eye-catching *tissue mast cells* (top center). Mast cells, residents of connective tissue, are distinguishable from their myeloid analogues, blood basophils, by their large size, round lavender nuclei, and compact coiffures of metachromatic granules. Collectively lymphocytes, plasma cells, and mast cells are like a gathering of scavengers and are known as *marrow injury cells*. That the marrow in **Figure 26-3** is severely hypoplastic can be inferred from the relative abundance of fat cells, but this interpretation lacks the histomorphic certainty of **Figure 26-1**.

Most aplastic anemias result from partial stem cell failure (*hypoplastic anemia*) in which hematopoietic marrow recedes unevenly, leaving behind foci or "hot pockets" of hyperplasia. **Figure 26-2** (×800) shows a desperate band of survivors struggling in a sea of fat. When the collective mass of red marrow is diminished but geographically scattered, marrow may reveal fatty tissue or dry taps on some specimens and atypical cellular marrow on others; this discontinuity underscores the need to obtain tissue sections in patients with suspected aplasia and, in some instances, to secure biopsies from both iliac crests. In the H&E–stained section portrayed in **Figure 26-2**, most of the clustered cells can be identified as erythroid cells by their agranular deep maroon cytoplasm and condensed nuclei, but the presence or absence of dysplasia cannot be ascertained readily. Their identity as a homogeneous enclave of polychromatophilic erythroblasts is luminously clear on a Wright-Giemsa–stained preparation (**Figure 26-4**, ×1,260). Aside from the monocyte (lower right) and a few lymphocytes, all of the cells in this field are late-stage erythroblasts, and most appear mildly megaloblastic, being somewhat large and showing tardy chromatin condensation. Uniform populations of erythroblasts of this description are found in hemolytic anemias and myelodysplastic syndromes, but in these settings erythropoietic elements fill the entire marrow cavity wall to wall. In aplastic anemia the scattered islands of surviving marrow are under intense pressure by the high levels of *erythropoietin* (EP) released from renal tubular cells during hypoxia. Remnant erythroid colonies are rushed into dysplastic maturation, and blood often contains large *stress reticulocytes*, macrocytes, and elevated levels of fetal hemoglobin.

In the United States and western Europe the annual age-specific new case incidence of aplastic anemia is 5 to 10 per million. About 50% of aplastic anemias have no known cause. Patients presenting with aplastic anemia should be questioned and explored carefully for evidence of causative factors. Among dose-dependent agents of myelotoxicity are ionizing radiations, drugs used in chemotherapy, and benzene. About 90% of secondary aplastic anemias occur as an unpredictable side effect of medication. At least 400 chemicals and drugs have been linked to unexpected idiosyncratic marrow failure, usually on circumstantial grounds. Notorious among these are chloramphenicol and several over-the-counter analgesics. Idiosyncratic aplasia, like the idiopathic process, is unresponsive to conventional therapies, yielding only to marrow transplantation. Systemic diseases predisposing to chronic marrow failure include *hepatitis C*, which accounts for more than 5% of aplastic cases requiring marrow transplantation, and endstage renal disease, in which the anemia responds to either renal transplantation or replacement of the renal hormone by *recombinant EP*. About 30% of aplastic anemias that appear in childhood are hereditary, the most common being a syndrome of defective DNA repair named *Fanconi's anemia*. Marrow transplanted from HLA-identical siblings can cure marrow failure but does not protect against neoplasms to which those patients afflicted with chromosomal instability are predisposed.

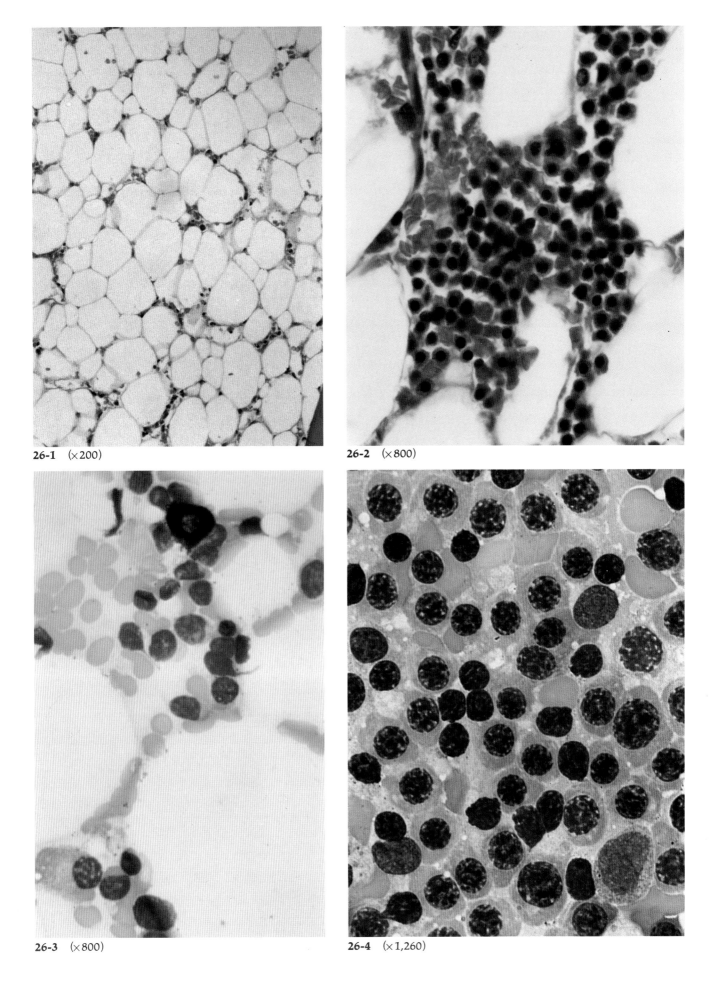

26-1 (×200)

26-2 (×800)

26-3 (×800)

26-4 (×1,260)

Figure 27. Myelophthisic Anemias. Infiltrative Myelopathy.

Infiltration of marrow by nonresident cells displaces native hematopoietic populations, interferes with regulation of blood cell formation, and disrupts the marrow : blood barrier. Because of the diminished hematopoietic tissue mass and deranged structure of the marrow, fewer cells are generated, and their release is often premature. The hallmarks in blood of marrow infiltration are teardrop-shaped red cells (**Figure 27-1**) and the inappropriate presence of erythroblasts (**Figure 27-2**) and early myeloid elements (**Figures 27-3** and **27-4**). Functionally, the marrow is hypoplastic, but because of the hasty liberation of numerous immature cells into the blood, the morphologic picture may be misjudged as evincing hematopoietic hyperactivity. The hematologic syndrome of (1) marrow infiltration with disruption of myeloid architecture, (2) appearance in the circulation of nucleated red cells, immature granulocytes, and giant platelets or chunks of megakaryocytes, and (3) presence of red cells with teardrop deformities is usually identified by the venerable expression *myelophthisic anemia*. An alternative term in wide use is *leukoerythroblastic anemia*, but the designation *infiltrative myelopathy* is recommended as more apt than either of these. When hematopoietic cells appear prematurely in the blood and in extramedullary nests, the imprecise term *myeloid metaplasia* is sometimes used. In parts of Europe, the myelophthisic syndrome, if caused by carcinomatosis and associated with thrombocytopenia and infiltrative splenomegaly, is known as the *syndrome of Weil (or Emile-Weil) and Clerc*. As nearly all myelophthisic anemias are caused by widespread diseases that involve microvasculature, it is not surprising that microangiopathic changes are commonly present and sometimes dominate the hematologic picture. The most prevalent sort of marrow infiltration is metastatic carcinoma, often with microvascular spread associated with microangiopathic changes and evidence of DIC. The primary sites of invasive carcinomas are most often the lungs, breast, prostate, or stomach. The next most frequent malignancies responsible for this syndrome are leukemias and lymphomas. The most common noncancerous cause of infiltrative myelopathy, miliary tuberculosis, is potentially curable and thus should always be searched for when myelophthisic changes are recognized. In immunodeficient patients, miliary tuberculosis often represents opportunistic infection by *Mycobacterium avium-intracellulare*. Other, relatively rare causes of disseminated lesions of the marrow are disseminated lupus erythematosus, the various granulomatoses, fungal and protozoan infections, osteomyelitis, lipid storage diseases, and proliferative disorders of macrophages (the "histiocytoses").

The chronic myeloproliferative disorder *idiopathic myelofibrosis*, alias *agnogenic myeloid metaplasia*, can be identical to infiltrative myelopathy in its effects on blood morphology. As with the myelophthisis of disseminated carcinoma, myelofibrosis is a common reason for the finding of a "dry tap" on attempted sternal aspiration. Inability to secure ample marrow from the sternum or iliac crest by needle aspiration is a clear indication for securing 1 or more marrow biopsies and thus for differentiating marrow fibrosis from any of the many causes of marrow infiltration cited previously.

As marrow cell replacement by tumor or fibrosis progresses, senior members of the stem cell hierarchy are dislodged into circulation and take up residence in the marrow-like microenvironment of the splenic red pulp. Hematopoietic colonization of splenic sinuses can become massive, particularly in patients with idiopathic myelofibrosis. Transplanted stem cells of all 3 major lineages may flourish and self-replenish in their exotic setting; when *extramedullary hematopoiesis* is anatomically appreciable, it is called *myeloid metaplasia*. At first, splenic hematopoiesis is confined to sinuses, but with time stem cells and their progeny spill into, inhabit, and distend the blind-ended cordal compartments. This traps and destroys megakaryocytes but does not cramp myeloid and erythroid elements, which continue to release their more nimble offspring. Escape of newly formed red cells from the chambers of their cordal nursery is slow and labored, however, and many cells are arrested for an hour or more while squeezing through the shingled apertures connecting cords to sinus outflow. During this mechanical trial, their cytoskeletons are rearranged to form tailed, tapered, or teardrop conformations. *Teardrop deformities* are the insignia of myeloinfiltrative disorders and the most apparent clue to a generic diagnosis (**Figure 27-1**, ×800). These "tell-tailed" forms often are accompanied by smaller numbers of contracted pyknocytes, as shown. The importance of the spleen in the pathogenesis of teardrop and allied forms is borne out by the fact that they disappear after splenectomy. Characteristically, reticulocyte levels are raised to about 4 to 6% (whether or not the patient is anemic), polychromatophils are oddly abundant, and nucleated red cells appear on the scene (**Figure 27-2**, ×1,260), suggesting violation of the marrow : blood barrier. Underscoring this interpretation is the finding of premature myeloid forms, which may be as young as the trespassing but normal promyelocyte shown in **Figure 27-3** (×2,000) but more often are represented by metamyelocytes (**Figure 27-4**, ×1,260). All 4 blood smears displayed on this page were obtained from patients with metastatic adenocarcinoma complicated by DIC. Thus, in each panel helmet cells or other schistocytes are conspicuous and platelets are quite sparse.

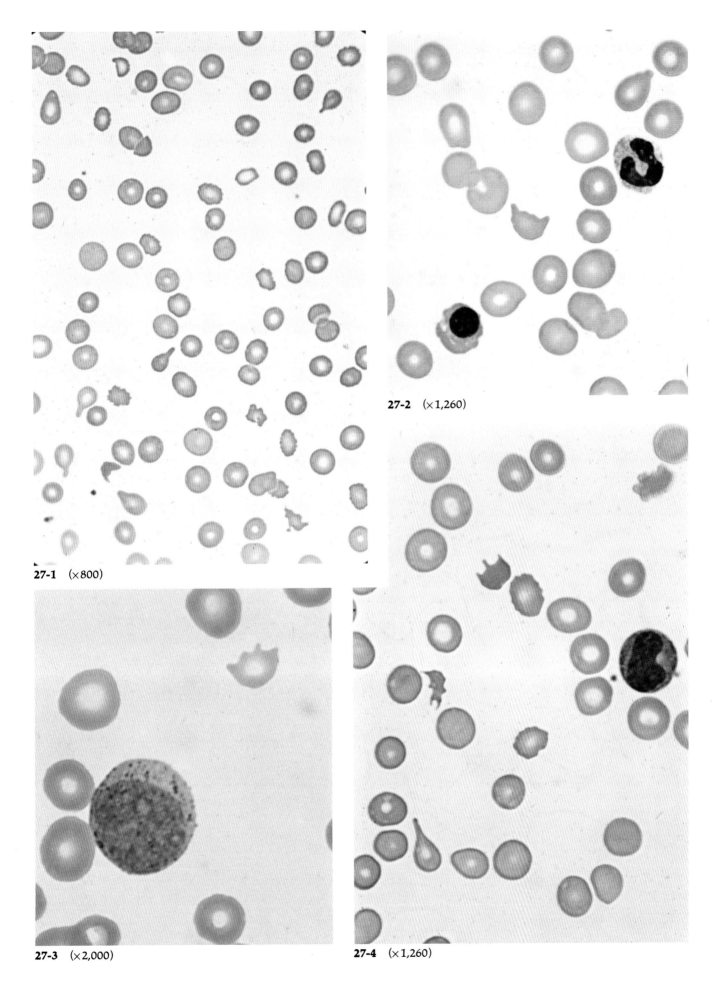

27-1　(×800)

27-2　(×1,260)

27-3　(×2,000)

27-4　(×1,260)

Figure 28. Metastatic Carcinoma

Scanning aspirates, touch preparations, or biopsies at low-power magnification is the most productive single ritual of marrow morphology. This not only steers the observer to well-spread, well-stained areas but also brings into view unnatural arrangements of cells. This practice is of paramount importance in the discovery of cell clusters, particularly when these are sparse or widely deployed, as in the thin yield of dry taps. Disorderly swarms of heaped-up cells, such as those shown in **Figure 28-1** ($\times 200$), command scrutiny. Clustering is the cachet of cancer. Marrow offers a favorable environment for implantation and spread of neoplastic cells. The number of macrophages in marrow is similar to that in liver, spleen, and lymphatics, but fewer are phagocytic: they are less hostile, less mobile, and less proliferative. Whereas infiltration of spleen by malignancy or disseminating tuberculosis usually is constrained, neoplastic cells and mycobacteria often invade the marrow unchecked. Even when the primary neoplastic lesion is undetectably small and before tumor dissemination elsewhere has been noted, the marrow cavity may be extensively invaded and myelophthisic changes may appear. Lesions of bone occur as a consequence of hematogenous spread into marrow, and "metastases to bone" actually represent colonization of bone marrow.

Metastatic carcinoma of bone marrow may assert its presence by inducing local pain, tenderness, or pathologic fractures. In some instances, the symptoms of anemia or signs of thrombocytopenia initiate investigations that lead to discovery of the myelopathic changes described in **Figure 27**, or to the finding of a dry tap on attempted needle aspiration of marrow. Often, attempted aspiration of infiltrated marrow evinces neither the usual pain nor appreciable quantities of marrow. Difficulty in obtaining sufficient marrow for cytologic and histologic examination can be circumvented if one does a needle biopsy at the outset. Certainly when the blood shows myelophthisic changes, needle biopsy is imperative. Risk from bleeding at the site of biopsy, even in thrombocytopenic purpura, is minimal; any persisting leakage of blood in severely thrombocytopenic patients is readily stanched by applying firm sterile pressure.

There are 4 nearly universal characteristics of metastatic cancer cells that differentiate them from resident marrow cells. (1) Invasive cells are usually larger than any marrow cells except megakaryocytes. (2) Tumor cells have a strong propensity for adhering to each other in mulberrylike aggregates or sheets. Even when marrow is so expertly spread on coverslips that few normal cells overlap, tumor cells will show clustering. (3) Individual tumor cells of each cluster or group usually differ considerably among themselves in size, shape, and intensity of staining. Most often, the cells stain overly blue or possess "unnatural" basophilic coloration. The cells are pleomorphic, nuclei are large, irregular, and sometimes multiple, and many cells are undergoing mitosis. (4) The cytoplasm of most tumor cells is diffusely and strangely granular and finely vacuolated and often has a webby look. Bluish wads of cytoplasmic debris are common, for, however dangerous, tumor cells are defective and frail. The heterogeneous chromatin patterns differ from the tidy patterns of normal, more regimental hematopoietic cells, and the nucleoli are often large, bizarre, and multiple.

The swarming appearance of sheets of poorly differentiated bronchogenic carcinoma cells is portrayed in **Figure 28-1**. A large cluster of anaplastic cells from the marrow of a woman with metastatic cancer of the breast is shown at a higher power ($\times 800$) in **Figure 28-2**. The pleomorphism is striking: no 2 cells look alike, each differing to some extent from the rest in nuclear size, shape, hue, and stage of chromatin condensation. The cytoplasm is equally heterogeneous, varying in amount from inapparent to plentiful, in complexion from smooth to vacuolated or granular, and in disposition from circumferential to segmentary. Metastatic cells are large as a rule, but there are exceptions. When tumor cells are about 12 to 16 μm in diameter, particularly if they are homogeneous and have round nuclei, they can simulate cells of acute lymphatic leukemia (ALL) or lymphocytic lymphoma. This similitude is demonstrated by cells from the marrow of a child with neuroblastoma (**Figure 28-3**, $\times 800$). Individually, many of these resemble the undifferentiated cells of childhood ALL, and several could easily be taken for young plasma cells. The cells are clearly of 1 cell type and thus represent a cluster. So large a cluster of any cell line in marrow can only mean that the cells are neoplastic. The cells are arranged in syncytial or arcuate arrays; in the rosette of 6 cells at the center of the figure, the blending of cytoplasm at their common junction is suggestive of neuroblastoma. Presence of rosette clusters involving several dozen cells grouped concentrically around a featureless blue-gray cytoplasmic "mush" more than 100 μm across is pathognomonic. If the anaplastic hemangioendothelioma cells clustered in **Figure 28-4** ($\times 800$) were not so huge, they would somewhat resemble neuroblastoma cells. Like them, these anaplastic cells adhere to each other (and not to such noncancerous cells as the neutrophil at the right of the figure); and like them, these cells contain many small vacuoles. They also tend to be spindle-shaped and polyploid, and there is a hint of geometric grouping, although too disorganized to suggest rosettes. It takes but a glance to recognize the malevolent nature of these malignant invaders.

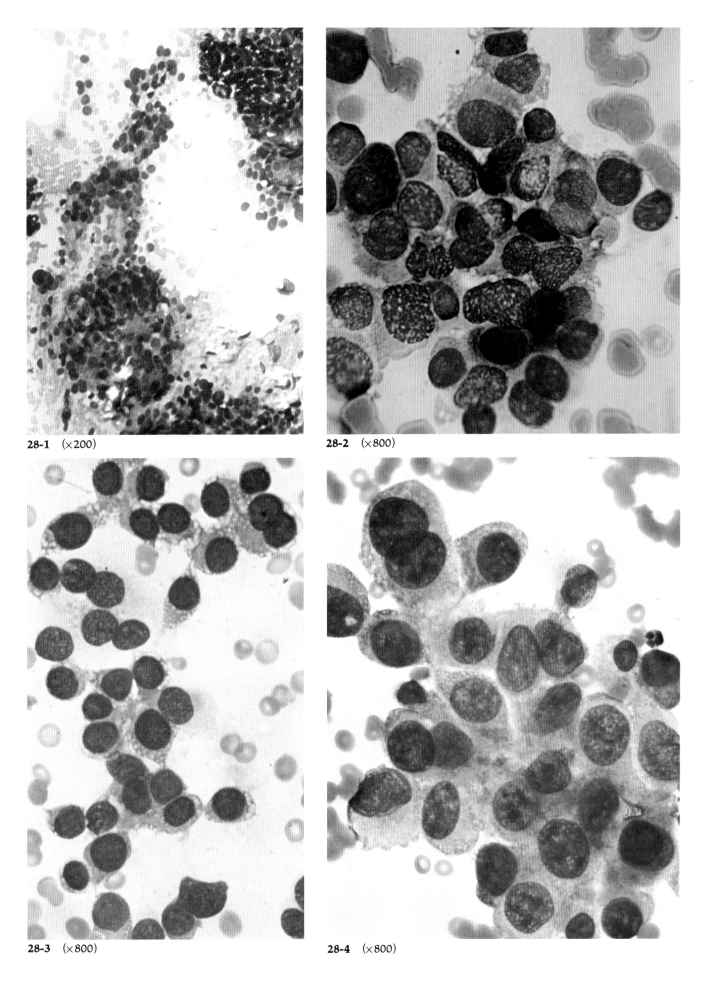

28-1 (×200)

28-2 (×800)

28-3 (×800)

28-4 (×800)

Bibliography

Megaloblastic Anemias

Amos RJ et al: Prevention of nitrous oxide-induced megaloblastic changes in bone marrow using folinic acid. Br J Anaesth 56 : 103, 1984

Babior BM and Stossel TP: Hematology. A Pathophysiological Approach, 2nd ed. New York, Churchill Livingstone, 1990

Baram J et al: Effect of methotrexate on intracellular folate pools in purified myeloid precursor cells from normal human bone marrow. J Clin Invest 79 : 692, 1987

Carethers M: Diagnosing vitamin B_{12} deficiency, a common geriatric disorder. Geriatrics 43 : 89, 1988

Chanarin I: The Megaloblastic Anemias, 3rd ed. Oxford, Blackwell Scientific Publications, 1990

Herbert V: Making sense of laboratory tests of folate status: folate requirements to sustain normality. Am J Hematol 26 : 199, 1987

Hoffbrand AV and Pettit JE: Chapt 3, in Clinical Hematology Illustrated. An Integrated Text and Color Atlas. London, Gower Medical Publishing Ltd, 1987

Jandl JH: in Cecil-Loeb Textbook of Medicine, 13th ed, Beeson PB and McDermott W, Eds. Philadelphia, WB Saunders Company, 1971

Kass L: Pernicious Anemia. Philadelphia, WB Saunders Company, 1976

Koistinen P et al: Hematopoietic and gastric uracil-DNA glycosylase activity in megaloblastic anemia and in atrophic gastritis with special reference to pernicious anemia. Carcinogenesis 8 : 327, 1987

Shields RW Jr and Harris JW: Subacute combined degeneration of the spinal cord and brain, in Current Therapy in Neurologic Disease–2, Johnson RT, Ed. Philadelphia, BC Decker Inc, 1987

Hypochromic Anemias

Babior BM and Stossel TP: Hematology. A Pathophysiological Approach, 2nd ed. New York, Churchill Livingstone, 1990

Bothwell TH et al: Chapt 2, in Iron Metabolism in Man. Oxford, Blackwell Scientific Publications, 1979

Bothwell TH and Charlton RW: A general approach to the problems of iron deficiency and iron overload in the population at large. Semin Hematol 19 : 54, 1982

Bottomley SS: Chapt 10, in Iron in Biochemistry and Medicine, II, Jacobs A and Worwood M, Eds. London, Academic Press, Inc (London) Ltd, 1980

Bottomley SS: Sideroblastic anaemia. Clin Haematol 11 : 389, 1982

Bowden DK et al: Different hematologic phenotypes are associated with the leftward ($-\alpha^{4.2}$) and rightward ($-\alpha^{3.7}$) α^+-thalassemia deletions. J Clin Invest 79 : 39, 1987

Brittenham GM et al: Magnetic-susceptibility measurement of human iron stores. N Engl J Med 307 : 1671, 1982

Cai S-P et al: A simple approach to prenatal diagnosis of β-thalassemia in a geographic area where multiple mutations occur. Blood 71 : 1357, 1988

Clark M et al: Interaction of iron deficiency and lead and the hematologic findings in children with severe lead poisoning. Pediatrics 81 : 247, 1988

Clegg GA et al: Ferritin: molecular structure and iron-storage mechanisms. Prog Biophys Mol Biol 36 : 53, 1980

Cook JD et al: Evaluation of the iron status of a population. Blood 48 : 449, 1976

Cook JD et al: Estimates of iron sufficiency in the US population. Blood 68 : 726, 1986

Cook JD and Lynch SR: The liabilities of iron deficiency. Blood 68 : 803, 1986

Erslev AJ and Gabuzda TG: Pathophysiology of Blood, 3rd ed. Philadelphia, WB Saunders, 1985

Halliday JW and Powell LW: Iron overload. Semin Hematol 19 : 42, 1982

Jandl JH: Chapt 6, in Blood: Textbook of Hematology. Boston, Little Brown and Company, 1987

Jandl JH: Chapt 7, in Blood: Pathophysiology. Boston, Blackwell Scientific Publications, Inc, 1991

Lozoff B and Brittenham GM: Behavioral aspects of iron deficiency. Prog Hematol 14 : 23, 1986

Orkin SH: Chapt 4, in The Molecular Basis of Blood Diseases, Stamatoyannopoulos G et al, Eds. Philadelphia, WB Saunders Company, 1987

Roberts GT and El Badawi SB: Red cell distribution widths in some hematologic diseases. Am J Clin Pathol 83 : 222, 1985

Seligman PA et al: Chapt 7, in The Molecular Basis of Blood Diseases, Stamatoyannopoulos G et al, Eds. Philadelphia, WB Saunders Company, 1987

Hemolytic Anemias

Agre P et al: Partial deficiency of erythrocyte spectrin in hereditary spherocytosis. Nature 314 : 380, 1985

Agre P and Parker JC, Eds: Red Blood Cell Membranes. New York, Marcel Dekker Inc, 1989

Aikawa M and Miller LH: Structural alteration of the erythrocyte membrane during malarial parasite invasion and intraerythrocyte development, in Malaria and the Red Cell. Ciba Foundation Symposium 94. London, John Wiley & Sons, Ltd, 1983

Andre R et al: Deux observations d'anemie hemolytique aique apres prise de phenyl-semi-carbazide. Remarques sur la poikilocytose et revue de la litterature. Nouv Rev Fr Hematol 5 : 431, 1965

Ash LR and Orikel TC: Atlas of Human Parasitology, 2nd ed. Chicago, ASCP, 1984

Babior BM and Stossel TP: Hematology. A Pathophysiological Approach, 2nd ed. New York, Churchill Livingstone, 1990

Benson LE et al: Entry of Bartonella bacilliformis into erythrocytes. Infect Immun 54 : 347, 1986

Bessis M: Corpuscles. Atlas of Red Cell Shape. Berlin, Springer-Verlag, 1974

Blaas P et al: Paroxysmal nocturnal hemoglobinuria. Enhanced stimulation of platelets by the terminal complement components is related to the lack of C8bp in the membrane. J Immunol 140 : 3045, 1988

Bluemke DA et al: The three-dimensional structure of sickle hemoglobin macrofibers, in Pathophysiological Aspects of Sickle Cell Vaso-Occulsion, Nagel RL, Ed. New York, Alan R. Liss, Inc, 1987

Bruce-Chwatt LJ: Essential Malariology, 2nd ed. London, William Heinemann Medical Books, 1984

Bull BS and Kuhn IN: The production of schistocytes by fibrin strands (a scanning electron microscope study). Blood 35 : 104, 1970

Bunn HF and Forget BG: Chapts 10 and 11, in Hemoglobin: Molecular, Genetic and Clinical Aspects. Philadelphia, WB Saunders Company, 1986

Burroughs SF et al: The population of paroxysmal nocturnal hemoglobinuria neutrophils deficient in decay-accelerating factor is also deficient in alkaline phosphatase. Blood 71 : 1086, 1988

Churchill WH and Kurtz SR, Eds: Transfusion Medicine. Boston, Blackwell Scientific Publications, 1988

Eaton WA and Hofrichter J: Hemoglobin S gelation and sickle cell disease. Blood 70 : 1245, 1987

Edelstein SJ: Structure of the fibers of hemoglobin S. Texas Rep Biol Med 40 : 221, 1980

Ham TH: Studies on destruction of red blood cells. I. Chronic hemolytic anemia with paroxysmal nocturnal hemoglobinuria: investigation of the mechanism of hemolysis, with observations on 5 cases. Arch Intern Med 64 : 1271, 1939

Jandl JH: Chapt 7, 9, and 13, in Blood: Textbook of Hematology. Boston, Little, Brown and Company, 1987

Jandl JH: Chapt 8, in Blood: Pathophysiology. Boston, Blackwell Scientific Publications, Inc, 1991

Kark JA et al: Sickle-cell trait as a risk factor for sudden death in physical training. N Engl J Med 317 : 781, 1987

Kaul DK et al: Vaso-occlusion by sickle cells: evidence for selective trapping of dense red cells. Blood 68 : 1162, 1986

Kulozik AE et al: Geographical survey of β^s-globin haplotypes: evidence for an independent Asian origin of the sickle-cell mutation. Am J Hum Genet 39 : 239, 1986

Mentzer WC and Wagner GM, Eds: The Hereditary Hemolytic Anemias. New York, Churchill Livingstone, 1989

Muller R and Baker JR: Medical Parasitology. Philadelphia, JB Lippincott Company, 1990

Murgo AJ: Thrombotic microangiopathy in the cancer patient including those induced by chemotherapeutic agents. Semin Hematol 24 : 161, 1987

Nagel RL, Ed: Genetically Abnormal Red Cells, Vols. 1 and II. Boca Raton, FL, CRC Press, Inc, 1988

Noguchi CT et al: Levels of fetal hemoglobin necessary for treatment of sickle cell disease. N Engl J Med 318 : 96, 1988

Palek J: Hereditary elliptocytosis, spherocytosis and related disorders: consequences of a deficiency or a mutation of membrane skeletal proteins. Blood Rev 1 : 147, 1987

Peters W and Killick-Kendrick R, Eds: The Leishmaniases in Biology and Medicine. London, Academic Press, 1987

Peters W and Gilles HM: A Colour Atlas of Tropical Medicine and Parasitology, 3rd ed. London, Wolfe Medical, 1989

Petz LD and Garraty G: Chapt 5, in Acquired Immune Hemolytic Anemias. New York, Churchill Livingstone, 1980

Petz LD and Swisher SN, Eds: Clinical Practice of Transfusion Medicine. New York, Churchill Livingstone, 1989

Pochedly C et al, Eds: Disorders of the Spleen. Pathophysiology and Management. New York, Marcel Dekker, Inc, 1989

Rosse WF: Interaction of complement with the red-cell membrane. Semin Hematol 16 : 128, 1979

Rosse WF: Autoimmune hemolytic anemia. Hosp Pract 20 : 105, 1985

Rosse WF: Clinical Immunohematology. Basic Concepts and Clinical Applications. Boston, Blackwell Scientific Publications, 1990

Serjeant GR: Sickle Cell Disease. New York, Oxford University Press, 1985

Valentine WN et al: Chapt 73, in The Metabolic Basis of Inherited Disease, 5th ed, Stanbury JB et al, Eds. New York, McGraw-Hill Book Company, 1983

Waugh RE and Agre P: Reductions of erythrocyte membrane viscoelastic coefficients reflect spectrin deficiencies in hereditary spherocytosis. J Clin Invest 81 : 133, 1988

Weatherall DJ: Common genetic disorders of the red cell and the 'malaria hypothesis.' Ann Trop Med Parasitol 81 : 539, 1987

Weinstein L: Preeclampsia/eclampsia with hemolysis, elevated liver enzymes, and thrombocytopenia. Obstet Gynecol 66 : 657, 1985

Wernsdorfer WH and McGregor I, Eds. Malaria: Principles and Practice of Malariology. Edinburgh, Churchill Livingstone, 1988

Wolf BC and Neiman RS: Disorders of the Spleen. Philadelphia, WB Saunders Company, 1989

Zail S: Clinical disorders of the red cell membrane skeleton. CRC Crit Rev Oncol Hematol 5 : 397, 1986

III. Nonneoplastic Disorders of White Cells

Reaction to Bacterial Infection

Figure 29. Bacterial Infection. Disseminated Tuberculosis. Marrow Necrosis.

Three changes in neutrophil morphology signal bacterial infection: *toxic granulation*, *Döhle bodies*, and *vacuolation* (**Figures 29-1** through **29-4**). The toxic band form and a segmented neutrophil bearing a pair of Döhle bodies in **Figure 29-1** (×1,500) represent 2 of the earliest and truest trademarks of sepsis. Infection by pyogenic organisms usually elicits a healthy neutrophilia within hours, reflecting a cytokine-driven outpouring of granulocyte reserves from the marrow. In the haste of mobilization, neutrophils—the infantry of host defense—burst into the bloodstream still laden with coarse purple (azurophilic) primary granules (**Figure 29-2**, ×2,000). Persistence of abundant primary granules in neutrophils connotes rushed maturation in response to alien intruders, for in the leisure of peacetime, primary granules are phased out during myeloid maturation and gradually are replaced by the smaller pink freckles of secondary (specific) granules. Primary granules are lysosomes, repositories of hydrolytic enzymes, antibiotic "defensins," and peroxidase. Toxic neutrophils are prepared for war. Döhle bodies, 2 of which are visible in the segmented neutrophil in **Figure 29-1**, are another marker of precipitous cytokinetics. Döhle bodies are faint oblong or comma-shaped patches that stain clear cerulean blue and tend to locate near the periphery of neutrophil cytoplasm without disturbing its contour. Composed of puddles of dissolving endoplasmic reticulum, Döhle bodies are often indistinct and are easily overlooked during cursory examination, but presence of these blue blotches is a remarkably specific indication of infection.

During severe or systemic infection, primary granules implode within phagosomal cisterns, leaving behind clear holes that coalesce into vacuoles. Discovery of numerous vacuoles (and especially of microorganisms within vesicular chambers) signifies overwhelming septicemia and deteriorating neutrophil function. More often, neutrophils and band forms can be found that are nearly degranulated, show lucent wounds, and have vague, irregular margins (**Figure 29-3**, ×2,000). Most of its toxic granules lysed, this valiant but failing band form contains a faint Döhle body at lower left. Protruding from its upper aspect is a broad, pale blue, glassy protuberance; this represents an advancing sticky *lamellipod* and signifies directed locomotion (chemotaxis). In crawling toward their quarry, neutrophils agitated by chemoattractants commonly display a single lamellipod anteriorly. This foot process is much larger and paler than Döhle bodies and extends beyond the general contour of the cell. This degranulated cell is still limping toward the enemy, attesting to the fact that neutrophils are suicide troops; in fulfilling their mission they are expendable and, when amassed, are converted ignominiously to pus.

Splenectomized or hyposplenic patients are vulnerable to first-encounter infections by encapsulated bacteria, and emergence of toxic neutrophils may herald onset of devastating septicemia. The "toxic poly" in **Figure 29-4** (×2,000) is surrounded by several harmless but telltale anomalies characteristic of splenic hypofunction. Pappenheimer bodies are particularly numerous in the red cell adjacent to the right aspect of the granulocyte. The bold black inclusion in the large polychromatophil at upper left is a Howell-Jolly body. A "giant platelet" is lurking at the upper right.

Like those of neutrophils, the granules of eosinophils also "explode" when exposed to noxious (usually immunogenic) substances, as exemplified by the 3 moth-eaten cells in **Figure 29-5** (×2,000). Note that these cells in blood from a patient with iodide sensitivity are most extensively degranulated (or vacuolated) at their outer margins.

In certain situations, the myeloid response to infection is highly proliferative so that, in addition to the 3 cytologic indicators of infection, granulocytopoiesis may become so brisk that the blood appears leukemoid. A response is termed *leukemoid* either when the white count has increased beyond about 30,000 per μl or when there is a pronounced shift toward immaturity. During vigorous myeloid responses, some metamyelocytes and a few myelocytes may appear in the blood. Rarely, promyelocytes also emerge, but the finding of myeloblasts should always be presumed to signify myelogenous leukemia. Exceptions to this rule are encountered now and then in patients with severe disseminated tuberculosis, especially those heavily infected individuals who show myelophthisic changes, develop morbid neutropenia, and respond histologically to infiltration of acid-fast bacilli by manifesting *marrow necrosis*. As shown in **Figure 29-6** (×800), an immunocompromised patient gravely ill with *disseminated miliary necrosis* was unable to form protective granulomas in reaction to the swarming bacilli and displayed instead punctate necrosis of the marrow. Note the nests of vacuolated cellular debris admixed with ghostly pink remnants of granulocytes, with apparent sparing of the erythroblasts. Ziehl-Neelsen staining revealed sheets of invading tubercle bacilli in this patient's marrow. The mortality in such patients is very high despite appropriate therapy.

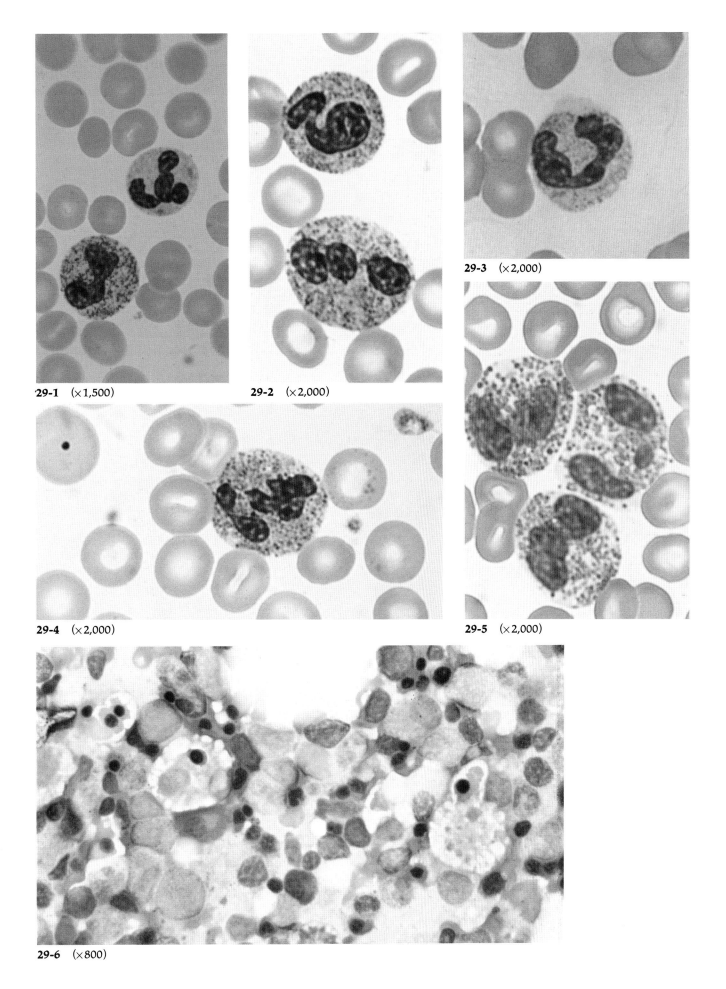

29-1 (×1,500)

29-2 (×2,000)

29-3 (×2,000)

29-4 (×2,000)

29-5 (×2,000)

29-6 (×800)

Inherited Morphologic Anomalies of Leukocytes

Figure 30. Pelger-Huët Anomaly. May-Hegglin Anomaly. Chediak-Higashi Syndrome. Hereditary Giant Neutrophilia. Alder-Reilly Anomaly.

Of the dozen or so hereditable deformities affecting 1 or all varieties of leukocytes, most are rare and all but 2 or 3 are harmless traits. Hereditary leukocyte aberrations, by convention, have been lumped together as anomalies, even though the *Chediak-Higashi syndrome* is often lethal in early life, the *May-Hegglin anomaly* may entail thrombocytopenic bleeding, and *Alder-Reilly granulations* often denote a serious metabolic disorder. **Figure 30-1** (×1,500) shows the 2 characteristic features of the *Pelger-Huët anomaly:* the pince-nez appearance of the bilobate nuclei and excessively coarse clumping of chromatin. In this benign dominant disorder, which has an incidence at birth of 200 per million, nuclear segmentation of the granulocytes is arrested in most cells (about 80%) at the 2-lobe level. Accordingly, there is a predominance of cells with twin, joined, plump nuclei resembling spectacles or dumbbells, admixed with a smaller number that possess an unlobulated oblong or peanut-shaped nucleus. In the few known homozygous individuals, all nuclei are round or pomegranate-shaped. The *pseudo–Pelger-Huët anomaly* is often acquired in the course of acute or chronic myelogenous leukemia and is a premonitory finding in myelodysplastic syndromes. The pseudo–Pelger-Huët anomaly may also be induced reversibly by cytotoxic agents. The acquired nuclear aberration can be differentiated from the constitutional form by 3 features: (1) among pseudo–Pelger-Huët cells, bilobate or pince-nez nuclear forms are in the minority; (2) there is a much higher percentage of normal, 3-lobed granulocytes than is found in the Pelger-Huët anomaly; and (3) pseudo–Pelger-Huët anomalous cells are usually found in the company of immature or leukemic cells.

The blood smear in **Figure 30-2** (×2,000) is from a patient with the *May-Hegglin anomaly*. This comparatively benign state is transmitted through an autosomal dominant gene and is characterized by (1) large abnormal Döhle bodies in all granulocytic cell types, including monocytes; (2) poorly granulated giant platelets; and (3) variable thrombocytopenia that may cause purpura. Some affected individuals have persisting leukopenia and predilection toward infection. Diagnosis depends on recognition that Döhle bodies are present in most granulated blood cells and in nearly all neutrophils. As exemplified by the 3-lobed neutrophil in **Figure 30-2**, the Döhle body of May-Hegglin type may be indistinguishable from that of infection, but most inclusions of May-Hegglin type are larger, more intensely blue, rounder and more sharply defined, and more numerous. In addition, the majority of May-Hegglin Döhle bodies are not peripherally placed but are disposed at random within the granulocyte, frequently ensconced between lobes of the cell nucleus. Toxic granulation and cytoplasmic vacuolation are not found in the May-Hegglin anomaly unless an infectious disorder is superimposed. Confirmation that the neutrophil in **Figure 30-2** is of the May-Hegglin type is provided by the presence of a giant platelet, almost the size of a red cell.

The *Chediak-Higashi* (or *Chediak-Steinbrinck-Higashi*) *syndrome* (congenital gigantism of peroxidase granules) is a rare, eventually fatal, inborn disorder, transmitted through autosomal recessive genes and marked by aggregation and gigantism of the granular structures of nearly all body cells. Among the most conspicuous of the early morbid changes are the following: partial oculocutaneous albinism with photophobia, nystagmus, peripheral neuropathy, and silvering of the hair; recurrent pyogenic infections; pancytopenia, often with thrombocytopenic purpura; progressive hepatosplenomegaly and lymphadenopathy; and ultimately, a sinister "accelerated phase" of widespread tissue infiltration by transformed lymphocytes. This lymphomalike phase is attributed to granular coalescence in NK cells, impairing their antiviral activity; this renders patients highly vulnerable to infection by transforming viruses such as Epstein-Barr virus. The diagnosis is easily made by examining blood or marrow smears, wherein most cell lines display gigantic primary granules. The neutrophil in **Figure 30-3** (×2,000) contains numerous enlarged primary-type granules arranged loosely as rosarylike strands of beads. Granular coalescence is more startling in lymphocytes (**Figure 30-4**, ×2,000). Even larger, solitary megagranules appear in many monocytes. Erythroid cells, on the other hand, show smaller and fewer granules, and megakaryocytes and platelets appear unaffected.

Several rare, dominantly inherited benign anomalies of neutrophils feature an increase in their size, in the degree of nuclear segmentation, or in ploidy. *Hereditary hypersegmentation of neutrophil nuclei,* in which at least 10% of neutrophils have 5 or more lobes, is harmless and rare. Also rare is *hereditary giant neutrophilia* (**Figure 30-5**, ×2,000), in which 1 to 2% of neutrophils are nearly twice normal in size, are tetraploid in DNA content, and often show evidence of nuclear twinning (so-called twinning deformity). Although most commonly there are 2 mirror-image sets of lobes, numbering from 3 to 5 segments each, there may be only 2 large potato-shaped nuclei in a single giant neutrophil. Giant neutrophils should not be confused with hypersegmented cells of megaloblastic anemias, wherein twinning or mirror-image patterns are not seen and the abnormal cells are only slightly enlarged. Neutrophil twinning may occur as an acquired anomaly in acute myelogenous leukemia and during therapy with alkylating and stathmokinetic agents.

A group of benign disorders marked by large and numerous reddish purple cytoplasmic granules in granulocytes, monocytes, and lymphocytes are cataloged under the heading *Alder-Reilly anomaly*. The intense, magenta hue of these multitudinous Alder-Reilly granulations is shown in **Figure 30-6** (×2,000) in both a neutrophil and a monocyte, and in **Figure 30-8** (×2,000) in another neutrophil. **Figure 30-7** (×2,000) shows the red-purple granulations, many having halos, of an affected lymphocyte. The abundance of red granules, particularly in marrow cells, the sheer number and size of the granules, the absence of Döhle bodies and vacuoles, and the prominent granulations in monocytes and lymphocytes provide ample criteria for distinguishing the Alder-Reilly anomaly from toxic granulation. Alder-Reilly granulations are not cytopathic but are indicators of 1 or another of the profound constitutional disturbances known as *mucopolysaccharidoses*. Among these are Hurler's syndrome, Hunter's syndrome, and polydystrophic dwarfism (Maroteaux-Lamy's syndrome).

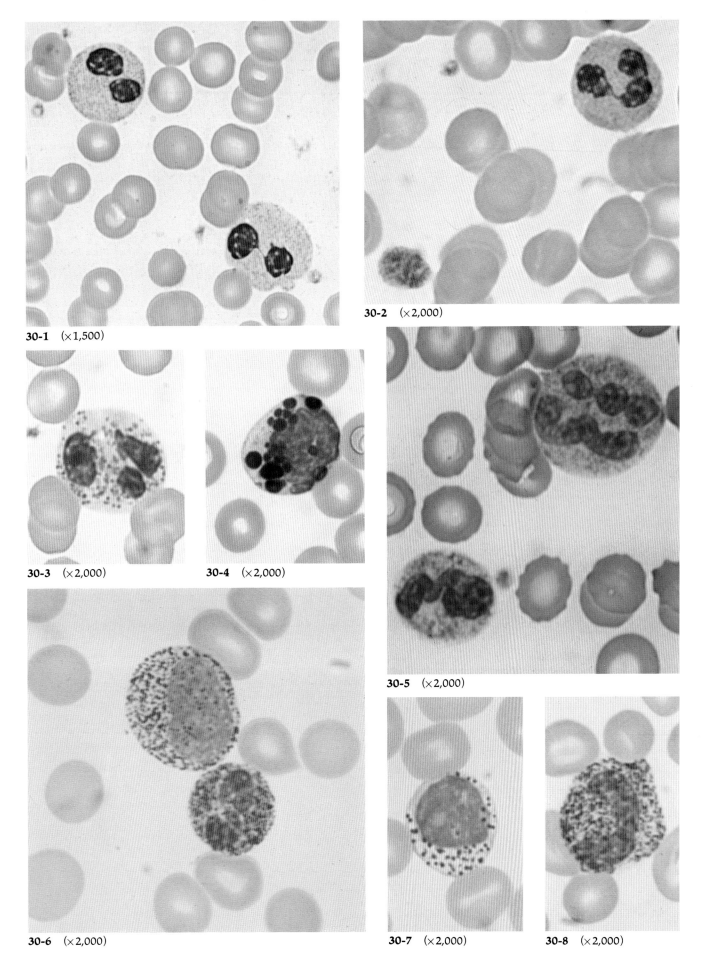

30-1　(×1,500)

30-2　(×2,000)

30-3　(×2,000)

30-4　(×2,000)

30-5　(×2,000)

30-6　(×2,000)

30-7　(×2,000)

30-8　(×2,000)

Inherited Morphologic Anomalies of Leukocytes　**71**

Bibliography

Aznar J and Vaya A: Homozygous form of the Pelger-Huet leukocyte anomaly in man. Acta Haematol (Basel) 66 : 59, 1981

Babior BM and Stossel TP: Hematology. A Pathophysiological Approach, 2nd ed. New York, Churchill Livingstone, 1990

Boxer LA and Smolen JE: Neutrophil granule constituents and their release in health and disease. Hematol Oncol Clin North Am 2 : 101, 1988

Cawley JC and Hayhoe FGJ: The inclusions of the May-Hegglin anomaly and Dohle bodies of infection: an ultrastructural comparison. Br J Haematol 22 : 491, 1972

Curnutte JT: Chronic granulomatous disease: clinical and genetic aspects, in Lehrer RI et al: Neutrophils and host defense. Ann Intern Med 109 : 127, 1988

Davidson WM et al: Giant neutrophil leukocytes: an inherited anomaly. Br J Haematol 6 : 339, 1960

Davidson WM: Inherited variations in leukocytes. Semin Hematol 5 : 255, 1968

Davis WC and Douglas SD: Defective granule formation and function in the Chediak-Higashi syndrome in man and animals. Semin Hematol 9 : 431, 1972

Dawborn JK and Cowling DC: Disseminated tuberculosis and bone marrow dyscrasias. Australas Ann Med 10 : 231, 1961

Ebina T et al: Time-lapse microcinematographic analysis of the natural cytotoxicity of murine lymphocytes: morphology of living natural killer [NK] cells. Microbiol Immunol 26 : 1095, 1982

Godwin HA and Ginsburg AD: May-Hegglin anomaly: a defect in megakaryocyte fragmentation? Br J Haematol 26 : 117, 1974

Groover RV et al: The genetic mucopolysaccharidoses. Semin Hematol 9 : 371, 1972

Grossi CE et al: Expression of the Chediak-Higashi lysosomal abnormality in human peripheral blood lymphocyte subpopulations. Blood 65 : 837, 1985

Haliotis T et al: Chediak-Higashi gene in humans. I. Impairment of natural-killer function. J Exp Med 151 : 1039, 1980

Hamilton RW et al: Platelet function, ultrastructure, and survival in the May-Hegglin anomaly. Am J Clin Pathol 74 : 663, 1980

Hughes JT et al: Leukaemoid reactions in disseminated tuberculosis. J Clin Pathol 12 : 307, 1959

Jandl JH: Chapt 19, in Blood: Textbook of Hematology. Boston, Little, Brown and Company, 1987

Klein M et al: Chediak-Higashi gene in humans. II. The selectivity of the defect in natural-killer and antibody-dependent cell-mediated cytotoxicity functions. J Exp Med 151 : 1049, 1980

Larrocha C et al: Hereditary myeloperoxidase deficiency: study of 12 cases. Scand J Haematol 29 : 389, 1982

Lusher JM and Barnhart MI: Congenital disorders affecting platelets. Semin Thromb Hemost 4 : 123, 1977

Marmont AM et al: Chapter 10, in Atlas of Blood Cells: Function and Pathology, vol. 1, Zucker-Franklin D et al, Eds. Milan, Edi. Ermes s.r.l., 1988

McCall CE et al: Lysosomal and ultrastructural changes in human "toxic" neutrophils during bacterial infection. J Exp Med 129 : 267, 1969

Medd WE and Hayhoe FGJ: Tuberculous miliary necrosis with pancytopenia. Q J Med 24 : 351, 1955

Parry MF et al: Myeloperoxidase deficiency: prevalence and clinical significance. Ann Intern Med 95 : 293, 1981

Pearson HA and Lorincz AE: A characteristic bone marrow finding in the Hurler syndrome. Pediatrics 34 : 280, 1964

Peterson L et al: Mucopolysaccharidosis type VII. A morphologic, cytochemical, and ultrastructural study of the blood and bone marrow. Am J Clin Pathol 78 : 544, 1982

Rausch PG et al: Immunocytochemical identification of azurophilic and specific granule markers in the giant granules of Chediak-Higashi neutrophils. N Engl J Med 298 : 693, 1978

Roder JC et al: The Chediak-Higashi gene in humans. III. Studies on the mechanisms of NK impairment. Clin Exp Immunol 51 : 359, 1983

Rook GAW: Role of activated macrophages in the immunopathology of tuberculosis. Br Med Bull 44 : 611, 1988

Royer HD and Reinherz EL: T lymphocytes: ontogeny, function, and relevance to clinical disorders. N Engl J Med 317 : 1136, 1987

Siegert E et al: Homozygotic Pelger-Huet anomaly. Kinderarztl Prax 51 : 164, 1983

Skendzel LP et al: The Pelger anomaly of leukocytes: forty-one cases in seven families. Am J Clin Pathol 37 : 294, 1962

Twomey JJ and Leavell BS: Leukemoid reactions to tuberculosis. Arch Intern Med 116 : 21, 1965

Virelizier J-L et al: Reversal of natural killer defect in a patient with Chediak-Higashi syndrome after bone-marrow transplantation. N Engl J Med 306 : 1055, 1982

White JG and Clawson CC: The Chediak-Higashi syndrome: the nature of the giant neutrophil granules and their interactions with cytoplasm and foreign particulates. I. Progressive enlargement of the massive inclusions in mature neutrophils. II. Manifestations of cytoplasmic injury and sequestration. III. Interactions between giant organelles and foreign particulates. Am J Pathol 98 : 151, 1980

Withers KL: Leukaemoid reactions in disseminated nonreactive tuberculosis: a review of the literature with report of a case. Med J Aust 2 : 142, 1964

Young JD-E and Cohn ZA: Cell-mediated killing: a common mechanism? Cell 46 : 641, 1986

Zieve PD et al: Vacuolization of the neutrophil: an aid in the diagnosis of septicemia. Arch Intern Med 118 : 356, 1966

IV. The Leukemias

Hematopoietic Malignancies

Figures 31 through 45. Introduction to Leukemias

Leukemias and lymphomas are cancers arising from unregulated clonal proliferation of hematopoietic stem cells. Individual cells generated by malignant clones are not programmed to differentiate fully or to function adequately. Malignant cells mature slowly and incompletely, their cell cycle time is prolonged, and most of these poorly differentiated cells survive longer than normal, arrested in their incompetence, mission unfulfilled. Leukemias and lymphomas are dangerous not because malignant cells divide too rapidly but because they never stop dividing. This pointless robotic growth and accumulation of tumor cells eventually crowds out and displaces normal hematopoietic residents in marrow and often threatens vital structures elsewhere. In leukemias, the most pervasive of cancers, accumulation of a lethal burden of tumor cells is usually achieved within 40 to 60 doubling times over a period ranging from 2 to 8 years. Each kind of leukemia and lymphoma has a different natural history, reflecting the cell type and stage at which differentiation was frozen. The importance of distinguishing between these heterogeneous diseases morphologically is that the correct choice of therapy is at stake.

Because all circulating white cells can be characterized as myeloid or lymphocytic, leukemias are categorized as either *myelogenous* or *lymphatic*. Lymphomas are clonal neoplasms of primary and secondary lymphoid tissue, and the taxonomy is more complex (see section VI, Lymphomas). Most lymphomas represent malignancies of cellular components of normal lymph nodes and are known as *non-Hodgkin's lymphomas*. Lymphomas displaying the talismanic Reed-Sternberg cell are known traditionally as *Hodgkin's disease*.

Acute myelogenous leukemia (AML) is a malignancy originating in marrow stem cells fully or partly committed to myeloid differentiation. If the underlying mutation is confined to colony forming units in granulocytes (CFU-Gs), the neoplastic proliferation leads to relatively pure accumulations of myeloblasts or promyelocytes. If the clonal lesion occurs 1 or 2 steps higher (earlier), all progeny of pluripotential stem cells are at risk, and the proliferative defect may be expressed by myeloid, monocytic, erythroid, or megakaryocytic lines, or combinations thereof. In any of its guises, AML proliferations suffocate normal marrow cells, and the end result is anemia, neutropenia, and thrombocytopenia, regardless of whether leukemic blast cells flood into the bloodstream. AML (sometimes called *acute nonlymphocytic leukemia*) comes in variant forms, each having unique morphology and some causing singular clinical manifestations. To aid prognosis and tailor therapy, AML has been classified morphologically into 7 subsets, and each has been given an *FAB* number (M1 through M7) by French-American-British luminaries. Collectively, AML in its variant forms is the most common entity, accounting for more than 50% of all leukemias and nearly 90% of acute leukemias. Most cases of AML occur de novo, but about 20% of patients experience a prefatory, often prolonged phase of trilineage marrow failure notable for cytologic dysplasias and hence called *myelodysplastic syndrome*. Used prospectively, the alternative term *preleukemia* must be considered conjectural, for fewer than half of patients presenting with myelodysplasia ever develop leukemia.

Chronic myelogenous leukemia (CML), the most common of the *chronic myeloproliferative syndromes*, results from a derangement at the multipotential stem cell level and is manifested initially by perpetual overproduction of granulocytes and their precursors. The cytogenetic hallmark of CML is the small but celebrated Philadelphia (Ph) chromosome, the minute product of a 9;22 translocation. CML is characterized by a mysteriously preordained triphasic course consisting of a long chronic phase, an interlude of acute transformation, and a stormy finale known as *blast crisis.*

Acute lymphatic leukemia (ALL), alias *acute lymphoblastic leukemia*, is a clonal malignancy of the committed lymphopoietic stem cells of marrow and is responsible for about 10% of all leukemias. Most ALLs are neoplastic counterparts of normal B cell precursors, and the B cell ALL that has its peak incidence between ages 2 and 6 years (childhood ALL) may be remarkably amenable to chemotherapy. Older children and adults with the FAB L2 and L3 subsets of ALL have less sunny prospects and more complex clonal lesions, reflecting damage higher up the stem cell hierarchy. As in AML, marrow infiltration by leukemic blast cells chokes off formation of normal cells, and, regardless of blast levels in blood, patients present with anemia, thrombocytopenia, and infection.

Chronic lymphatic leukemia (CLL) and the less common *prolymphocytic leukemia* and *hairy cell leukemia* are clonal lymphoproliferative disorders usually of B cell lineage that afflict people during late adulthood. CLL, the most common of chronic leukemias, is a languid process marked by ceaseless propagation of immense numbers of normal-appearing but immunologically indolent lymphocytes. Amassment of lymphocytes in marrow, blood, and tissues can be curbed for many years in most patients by judicious and gentle use of chemotherapy, but the leukemic process sometimes transforms to more impetuous proliferations.

Figure 31. Myelodysplastic Syndromes

Myelodysplastic syndromes are insidious clonal disorders of marrow that derange all nonlymphoid hematopoietic cell lines and often transform eventually into AML. That myelodysplasia is commonly a prelude to AML has popularized the term *preleukemia,* an overstated foreboding considering that 60% of patients never progress to overt leukemia. Primary myelodysplasia begins as a puzzling anemia unresponsive to all hematopoietic nostrums—hence the nonce phrase *refractory anemia.* Evolution to pancytopenia points to trilineage marrow failure, but the malfunctioning marrow is paradoxically hypercellular. The first clue to this difficult diagnosis is discovery on blood smears of strange but recurrent anomalies of myeloid cells. **Figure 31-1** (×1,260) shows 3 of the most visible logos of myelodysplasia: *pseudo–Pelger-Huët anomalies,* nuclear : cytoplasmic dyssynchrony, and importunate myeloblasts. The 2 bilobed pelgeroid neutrophils bracketing center stage are ominous facsimiles of the harmless inborn anomaly displayed in **Figure 30-1**: the plump pairs of condensed, mirror-image lobes linked by thin chromatin strands complete the pince-nez simulation. Both immature myeloid cells at bottom show discordant maturation. The promyelocyte at bottom left is too small for its heavy cargo of reddish primary granules, and the cell at bottom right is a dwarf myelocyte. The myeloblast near the top (next to an agranular pelgeroid cell) is misshapen and contains an oversized, oddly angulated nucleolus. Red cells are also affected in this patient, showing an assortment of poikilocytic deformities.

All marrow cells are stigmatized by myelodysplasia, but the most grotesque disfigurements are found in megakaryocytes. In the top-to-bottom lineup shown in **Figure 31-2** (×1,260), the 4 deranged megakaryocytes are consecutively tetranuclear, trinuclear, binuclear, and mononuclear. Normally megakaryocyte nuclei undergo endoreduplication so that each diploid lobe is connected in series; megakaryocytes having separated nuclei are among the most conspicuous markers of myelodysplasia. Many doyens of dysplasia regard triple nuclei deployed in a *pawnball pattern* (at center) as the imprimatur of myelodysplastic syndromes.

Myelodysplastic processes are dominated by ineffective erythropoiesis and, early in the course, marrow space is overrun by clonal colonies of erythroblasts displaying megaloblastoid features reminiscent of those in nutritional megaloblastic anemias. At the center of **Figure 31-3** (×1,260) is a cluster of proerythroblasts, 4 of which are abnormally large and contain curdled chromatin, punctured in each cell by a suspiciously large and prominent nucleolus. These malignant-looking erythroblasts are surrounded by orbitals of offspring whose level of differentiation increases with distance from their forebears. As in nutritional megaloblastic anemias, the cumulative maturational defects and degree of nuclear : cytoplasmic dissociation are most striking in the most mature cells. The threesome at the lower right, for example, possess abundant polychromatophilic cytoplasm, but the nuclear chromatin is uncondensed and checkered. The rich erythroid cellularity of this field of marrow is deceptive, for most of the cells are ordained to die in situ of their flawed clonal kinetics. The hypercellularity of dysplastic marrow reflects accumulation of sickly cells incapable of vigorous replication. That these defective hematopoietic elements displace normally healthy cells represents a biological triumph of pathologic proliferation over physiologic differentiation. In this patient with refractory anemia and ringed sideroblasts (not shown), there was no indication of leukemic transformation. The few myeloid cells in this field show normal maturation.

On the basis of narrow morphologic criteria, 4 distinctive myelodysplastic syndromes have been sanctioned by FAB terminologists. Patients do not recover from *refractory anemia* (RA) and *refractory anemia with ringed sideroblasts* (RARS), but in only about 10% does the clonal disorder transform into AML. In patients with a worrisome excess of blasts in the marrow *(refractory anemia with an excess of blasts* [RAEB]*)* the likelihood of leukemic transformation approaches 50%, and when myeloblasts plus promyelocytes comprise more than 30% of marrow elements—or when over 5% of nucleated blood cells are myeloblasts—the patient is said to be "in transformation" to AML (RAEB-T). The marrow field shown in **Figure 31-4** (×1,260) is from a patient with RAEB who died several months later of AML. In this scene, the marrow space is being overgrown with a mixture of robust-appearing promyelocytes and lesser numbers of small dysplastic (dwarf) myeloblasts (right-center). In some patients with this morbid cytology, progression may be sidetracked or even stalled for months or years, but usually encroachment to this degree by promyelocytes and myeloblasts represents the preamble to AML. Unfortunately, blast cells that flourish in myelodysplastic syndromes are locked in a proliferative mode that defies most efforts at therapy. Despite the canonical weight placed on the FAB classification of myelodysplastic syndromes, in the authors' opinion more than 20% myeloblasts in marrow (expressed as a proportion of myeloid elements only) indicates leukemia and nothing less.

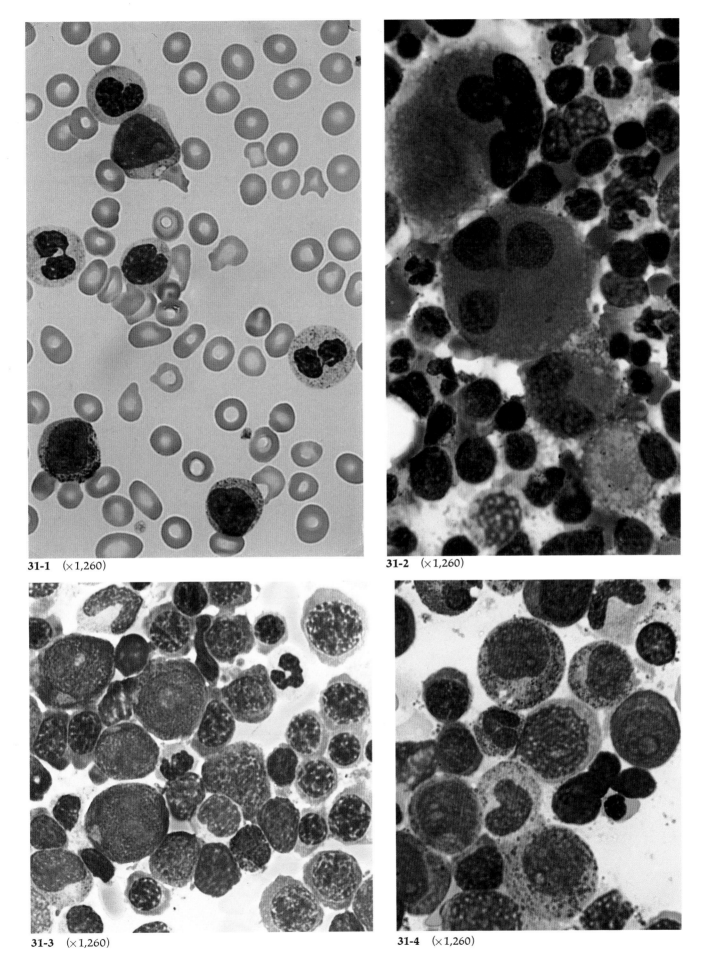

31-1 (×1,260)

31-2 (×1,260)

31-3 (×1,260)

31-4 (×1,260)

Acute Myelogenous Leukemia

Figure 32. Acute Myelogenous Leukemia without and with Maturation. Auer Rods.

Acute myelogenous leukemia too often is identified by what it is not: *acute nonlymphocytic leukemia*. AML comes in 7 variant forms, denoted M1 through M7, that ultimately share similar clinical features including a guarantee of death within several months if left untreated. In any of their many guises, AML myeloblasts accumulate in marrow because maturation is frozen at some transient stage of early differentiation. These hordes of undifferentiating, uncivilized, brutish blast cells dispossess the more orderly ranks of differentiating normal marrow cells. The result is anemia, neutropenia, and thrombocytopenia, and sooner or later the insensate overproduction of leukemic cells causes them to pour out into the bloodstream (**Figures 32-1** through **32-3**).

In AML of children and young adults, the underlying mutation usually is confined to committed stem cells (CFU-G or CFU-GM) and such "committed cell leukemias" may be chemocurable. In AML of later adulthood, the leukemic clone includes erythroid, megakaryocytic, and sometimes lymphoid lineage markers ("lineage infidelity"), indicating that the clonal defect is traceable to the multipotential stem cell level. In cellular as in human societies, infidelity is dangerous. Biphenotypic or multiphenotypic leukemias devolved from high-echelon stem cells can be exorcised only by ablation-and-rescue through marrow transplantation.

In AML without maturation, the primitive myeloblasts have the impersonal conformity of invading legions (**Figure 32-1**, ×2,000). The battalions of blasts shown here betray a lack of refinement and individuality characteristic of primitive cancer populations. Malignant myeloblasts vary considerably in shape but have a sinister homogeneity in coloration. Nuclear chromatin possesses a characteristic ground-glass texture, and nucleoli are pale and punched-out looking, unlike the bold marginated nucleoli of lymphoblasts. Although the numerous blasts in this blood smear (the patient had a white count of 160,000 cells/µl) look more like myeloblasts than lymphoblasts because of their ample, pale cytoplasm, soft-grained nuclear pattern, and overall violaceous hue, the cells are too undifferentiated for positive identification without use of special stains (see **Figure 33**). A clue to classification is the association with a dysplastic promyelocyte partly visible at the top.

In AML with partial maturation, the dominant M2 blast population displays primary granules, the more abundant cytoplasm has a bluer cast, and most nuclei are eccentric and show early evidence of chromatin clumping, however blotchy. The truest credentials authenticating the large blasts in **Figure 32-2** (×2,000) as myeloblasts are the long, red, needle-shaped cytoplasmic inclusions known as *Auer rods*. Auer rods are cylindrical stacks of dysplastic primary granules that fuse into splinter-shaped structures, which when numerous form characteristic crisscross arrangements. Their origin from coalescent primary (azurophilic) granules is attested by their staining for myeloperoxidase and for α-naphthol AS-D chloroacetate esterase. An indisputable marker for AML, Auer rods are found in most M2 and M4 variants, are particularly numerous in acute promyelocytic leukemia (M3), and sometimes appear in small numbers in acute monocytic leukemia (M5). They are not found in chronic myelogenous leukemia except very rarely during myeloid blast crisis. In M1 AML, Auer rods are scarce but

worth the effort of ferreting out, for their discovery in poorly differentiated leukemic cells certifies myeloid genealogy and affects choice of therapy.

In some patients with AML the myeloblasts are notable for their uneven size as well as their expanded numbers. Normal myeloblasts are uniformly styled in size and shape. Leukemic myeloblasts (and the dysplastic blasts of RAEB) are uniform in color (**Figure 32-1**) but often vary widely in size and design, as shown in **Figure 32-3** (×1,260). In this blood from a patient with an extremely high white count, about half the myeloblasts are unusually large and exhibit conspicuous multiple nucleoli of variable size. The half dozen smaller cells are *micromyeloblasts*, dwarf variants possessing scant, blue cytoplasm and tiny indistinct nucleoli. Were it not for the fineness of the nuclear chromatin of the micromyeloblasts and the deadly company they keep, these small members of the neoplastic clone might be mistaken for youthful lymphocytes. To affirm the diagnosis and exclude the remote possibility of a biclonal acute leukemia, use of special cytochemical stains is warranted.

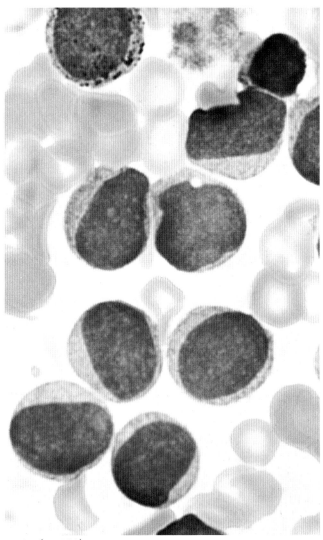

32-1 (×2,000)

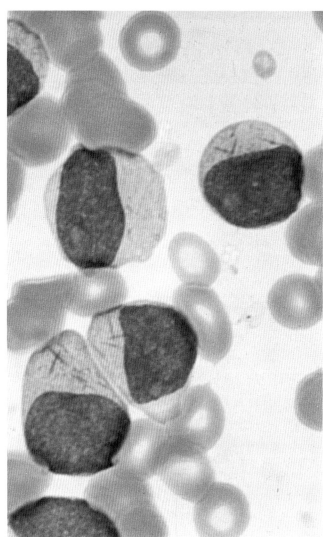

32-2 (×2,000)

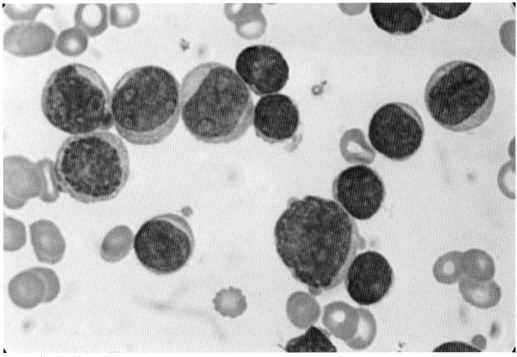

32-3 (×1,260)

Figure 33. Cytochemical Characteristics of Acute Leukemias

The cytologic type and lineage of acute leukemia blast cells can be recognized in nearly 90% of patients by use of conventional panoptic stains such as Wright-Giemsa. Valuable support in characterizing the kind of leukemia also comes from cellular associations. While viewing clusters of nondescript blast cells in marrow, discovery of intermixed promyelocytes and of myelodysplastic changes in neighboring cells undeniably points to a diagnosis of AML. Similarly, poorly differentiated blasts nested in colonies of immature lymphocytes can safely be accepted as lymphoblasts. The company-kept approach has its limits, however, for the least identifiable blasts in blood or marrow are often unaccompanied by kindred forms, particularly during explosive proliferations, and conventional criteria for distinguishing myeloid from lymphoid blasts may mislead. Small myeloblasts (micromyeloblasts) may resemble lymphoblasts, and large lymphoblasts with abundant cytoplasm, prominent nucleoli, and (rarely) cytoplasmic inclusions may be mistaken for myeloblasts. Selection of specific and appropriate therapy depends on correct identification of the enemy (blast cells), and for this purpose use of special *cytochemical stains* that demonstrate lineage-associated enzymes or metabolites is of paramount importance. A basic battery of cytochemical stains should be used in diagnosis of all acute leukemias. The most useful of these are *myeloperoxidase stain* and its operational backup, *Sudan black B* (**Figures 33-1** and **33-2**); *periodic acid–Schiff* (PAS) *reaction* (**Figures 33-3** through **33-5**); and stain for *nonspecific esterase activity* (**Figure 33-6**). In addition, immunophenotyping for cell antigen markers is of considerable value in diagnosis and classification of ALL (for which no specific cytochemical markers exist) and of the M7 variant of AML.

The rubric of myeloid cells is their enzyme-laden cargo of cytoplasmic granules, which distinguishes them from lymphoid cells. The large primary (nonspecific) granules of myeloid cells are rich in lysosomal peroxidase (myeloperoxidase), a vigorous enzyme that transfers hydrogen from various dye substrates to yield colorful deposits at the site of enzyme activity. The strongest, most aesthetically pleasing reaction color is the bold blue-green that lights up the stacked primary granules (Auer rods) in 4 of the myeloblasts shown in **Figure 33-1** (×2,000). Wright-Giemsa counterstaining emphasizes the dimensions of these inclusions, and green smudges of free, unpackaged peroxidase activity can be seen leaking into the cytoplasm of the blast at lower right. Presence of peroxidase positivity in more than 3% of blasts identifies the leukemia as of myeloid origin. Unfortunately, benzidine used as substrate in this illustration is a potential bladder carcinogen and has been replaced in most laboratories by the less emphatic dyes, diaminobenzidine (DAB), p-phenylene diamine, and 3-amino-9-ethylcarbazole, which yield hues ranging from dull gray to red-brown. Peroxidase activity is present at all stages of neutrophil development, in eosinophils, and (faintly) in monocytes, but is absent from erythroid cells and (by light microscopy) from megakaryocytes and platelets. A more sensitive and increasingly popular alternative to peroxidase stains is the lipophilic pigment, Sudan black B (**Figure 33-2**, ×2,000), which forms gray-to-black deposits in secondary as well as primary granules of neutrophils and their granular cousins. Hence the granules and Auer rods (see the thick black vertical bar in the cell at top center) show black spots, promyelocytes (below) are diffusely gray, and even neutrophils are blackened. For some reason, sudanophilia closely parallels peroxidase activity.

The PAS reaction, which stains carbohydrates (notably glycogen) red or pink, has little value as a lineage marker, for it colors most blood cells (except mature red cells) to some extent, being particularly rosy in neutrophils and platelets. Its value in acute leukemias lies in the pattern and context of staining. ALL lymphoblasts usually (not always) display either chunks (**Figure 33-3**, ×2,000) or heavy perinuclear granules (**Figure 33-4**, ×2,000) of red material, quite unlike the diffuse pink tinge or freckling sometimes seen in the M3, M4, or M5 variants of AML. "Block" patterns of PAS positivity are characteristic of ALL blasts but are not unique, being found occasionally in acute monocytic leukemia and occurring as a conspicuous diagnostic feature of *acute erythroleukemia* (**Figure 33-5**, ×2,000). Although stainable glycogen is sometimes found in thalassemic erythroblasts, normal erythroid cells are PAS-negative. In erythroleukemia (M6), variable red granularity is found in early erythroid precursors, and some of the more outré dysplastic proerythroblasts may display multiple chunks of deep carmine material. For grading intensity, compare the roseate neutrophils below with the spotted binucleated giant just above.

Cytochemical reactions for esterases using various artificial substrates permit distinction between myeloblastic and monoblastic leukemias, often a problematic matter when the acute monocytic leukemia (AMoL) blasts and promonocytes show only partial differentiation yet possess sudanophilic granules. The somewhat capricious *specific esterase* reaction using naphthol AS-D chloroacetate as substrate is usually positive (red) in nonspecific granules (including Auer rods) of myeloid precursors but not of monocytes. The more decisive *nonspecific esterase* using α-naphthyl butyrate as substrate actually is monocyte-specific (**Figure 33-6**, ×1,260), yielding either a blue or, as shown here, a rusty red hue, depending on the coupler. In this AMoL with partial differentiation (M5$_b$ variant), the more mature cleaved or curled-up nuclei stand out as negative-image cameos against the russet cytoplasm.

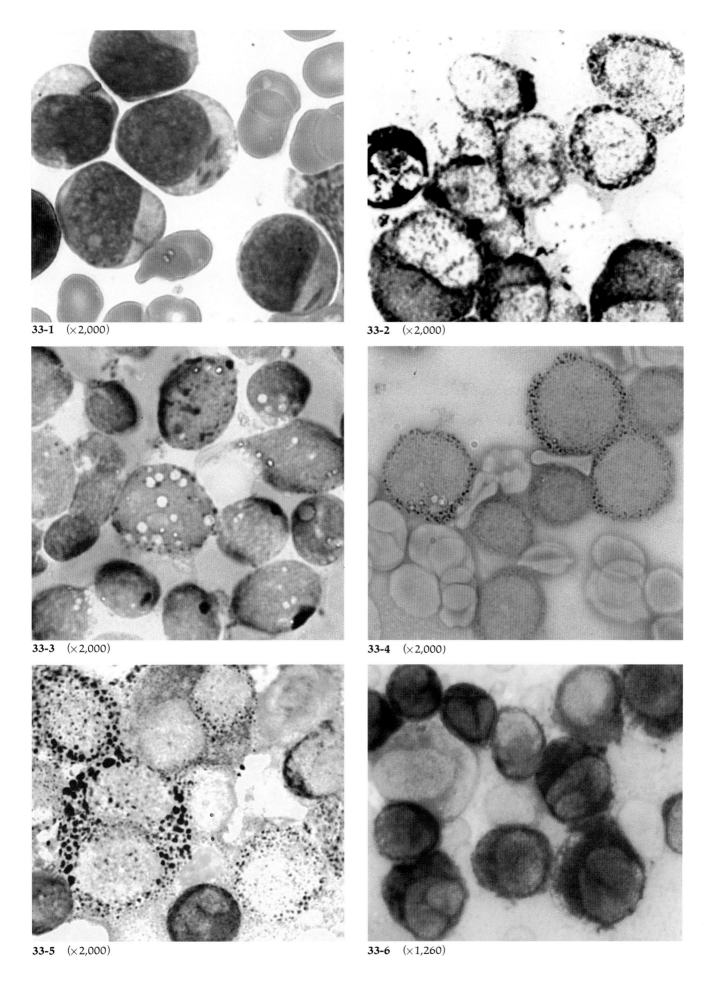

33-1 (×2,000)

33-2 (×2,000)

33-3 (×2,000)

33-4 (×2,000)

33-5 (×2,000)

33-6 (×1,260)

Figure 34. Marrow in Acute Myelogenous Leukemia. Oligoblastic Leukemia. Acute Promyelocytic Leukemia.

It cannot be overemphasized that AML is foremost a marrow disease, that in most patients morbidity results from dislodgment of normal marrow parenchyma by leukemic infiltrates, and that nearly one-third of patients present with low white counts and few blasts in the blood. During covert progression of AML, even as marrow function is being sabotaged extensively, typical cancer symptoms (unexplained weight loss, fever, night sweats) are unusual, and the first shadow of misfortune may be fortuitous discovery of 1 or more cytopenias associated with small numbers of myeloblasts. The canonical requirement for more than 5% myeloblasts in blood and 30% blasts in marrow to justify diagnosis of AML is ripe for revision, since "preleukemic" (RAEB-T) patients with 10 to 30% myeloblasts in marrow nearly always progress to frank AML. **Figure 34-1** (×800) gives a low-power view of marrow from a patient who for several months had had pancytopenia, minor myelodysplastic aberrations of myeloid cells, and low blood blast levels (1 to 5% of myeloid cells). Marrow aspirate at this juncture shows ample representation by both myeloid and erythroid elements, but about 15% of all marrow cells and nearly 30% of myeloid cells are myeloblasts, statistics sufficient for diagnosis of AML. The early natural course of de novo AML can be explosive, but in 20 to 30% of cases a smoldering battle for survival between normal and defective cell lines may wax and wane for months or, occasionally, years. This temporary standoff has generated elaborate terminology (*"myelodyssemantics"*), much of it incorporated in the FAB lexicon, but when marrow blasts are this numerous and show an ominous predilection to congregate in clusters, the preferred diagnosis (absent an outpouring of blasts into the bloodstream) is *oligoblastic leukemia*. Note in this field some myelodysplastic accompaniments of AML: megaloblastoid changes in erythroblasts and 2 agranular band forms.

Diagnosis of *acute promyelocytic leukemia* (APL or AML M3) is made when marrow contains more than 30% promyelocytes, regardless of the number of leukemic promyelocytes in blood. Ordinarily APL is the most diagnosable leukemia in the AML family because cytoplasm of the leukemic cells is stuffed with reddish primary granules, as exemplified in **Figure 34-2** (×800). Some of the larger promyelocytes look relatively normal, with lumpy nuclei (partly obscured by primary granules) and vague nucleoli. The majority of cells resemble myeloblasts in their dimensions and nucleoli but are so heavily freighted with variably colored granules that the tumor cells are termed *hypergranular promyelocytes*. Auer rods usually are numerous in APL cells, but if any are present in this field, they are lost in the profusion of gaily colored granules. In the few remnant neutrophils, note the dysplastic twinning and pelgeroid deformities. On closer view (**Figure 34-3**, ×2,000), the gaudy hypergranularity of malignant promyelocytes is stunning. Note that in the most heavily granulated cells, the dysplastic granules have an unusually dark red or magenta hue, whereas in others the granules have a more normal red-purple color. Several Auer rods are lurking in the small red-speckled cell near top center.

In 20% of APLs, the dysplastic primary granules are either barely evident or invisible by light microscopy (**Figure 34-4**, ×2,000), however abundant and apparent they may be on electron microscopy. A telltale feature of this morphological variant is that the well-exposed nucleus is often bilobate or even binuclear and nucleoli are unusually conspicuous. In the collection of bilobate *microgranular forms* arranged in **Figure 34-4**, the most characteristic is the cell at bottom left

showing 2 disconnected but partly overlapping and swivelled lobes. Note the artfully angular patterns formed by bundles of Auer rods in an otherwise "hypogranular" promyelocyte at the lower right.

It is essential that APL be recognized, for the multitudes of cytoplasmic granules, large and small, are laden with procoagulants that leak out of these malignant but fragile cells and trigger DIC. Of the FAB 7 family, APL is among the most responsive to chemotherapy, emphasizing the need for early diagnosis. In patients with confusing morphology diagnosis is certified by demonstrating the pathognomonic (15;17) translocation, although cytogenetic analysis is sometimes thwarted by the fuzzy chromosome morphology characteristic of leukemic promyelocytes.

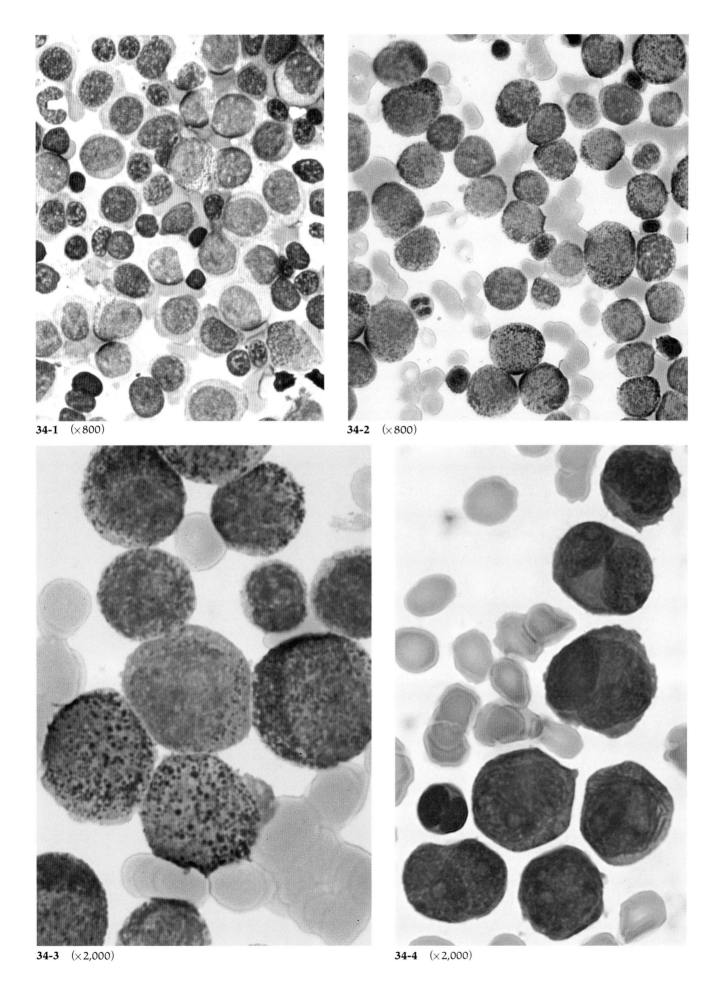

34-1 (×800)

34-2 (×800)

34-3 (×2,000)

34-4 (×2,000)

Figure 35. Acute Myelomonocytic Leukemia. Charcot-Leyden Crystal. Acute Monocytic Leukemia.

When, at first glance, marrow appears chock full of myeloblasts, but, on closer scrutiny, the infiltrate is found to be a disorderly mixture of cells having rounded, ameboid, or indented nuclei, *acute myelomonocytic leukemia* (AMML) should come to mind. In AMML (the M4 variant) both myeloblasts and monoblasts and their immediate descendants coexist in proportions ranging reciprocally from 20 to 80%. In **Figure 35-1** (×800) the prevailing cells are myeloblasts, moderately large, round violaceous cells with plump eccentric nuclei containing from 1 to 5 nonuniform, punched-out nucleoli. Nuclear chromatin is velvety, and the cytoplasm holds but a few refined granules (M1 properties). Intermixed among these classic myeloblasts is a population of darker, more contorted cells, many extending pseudopods and displaying nuclear notches, folds, clefts, and twists. These ameboid monoblasts are accompanied by small numbers of bluer promonocytes and a few well-differentiated, wrinkled, gray monocytes. Very few differentiating myeloid cells remain in evidence, among them an eosinophil myelocyte at left center and a pair of promyelocytes lurking at the upper left. The 2 lines of tumor cells in AMML are sibling products of a mutation at the CFU-GM branchpoint, but their relative numbers can vary vastly and confusingly between blood and marrow. Myeloblasts prefer to linger in marrow, while the more nimble monocytic forms slither off into circulation. The monocytoid leukemic cells in AMML stain strongly for nonspecific esterase but only weakly and unevenly, if at all, for peroxidase and Sudan black B. Myeloid components of this malignant melange react as expected to the standard myeloid marker stains, peroxidase and Sudan black B, although in immature blasts sudanophilia is the more dependable indicator. Myeloblasts react feebly for nonspecific esterase, but cytoplasm is colored bright red by stains for specific esterase (using naphthol AS-D chloroacetate as substrate), color intensity being a direct function of maturation. Single-step tinctorial techniques devised for simultaneous demonstration of nonspecific and specific esterases facilitate diagnosis of M4 variants of AML, but the distinction between red-brown and bright red is not as sharp or obvious as when two-stage red-blue complementary color couplers are employed.

A variant form of AMML that is unusually responsive to standard chemotherapy is notable for plentiful marrow eosinophils and a peculiar cytogenetic anomaly involving pericentric inversion of chromosome 16. The numerous eosinophils and eosinophil myelocytes congregated among the monocytoid blasts in marrow are laden with dysplastic granules, many or most of which are magenta-colored or strangely basophilic. Occasionally in this, the AML M4Eo variant, multicolored granules leaking from the neoplastic eosinophils fuse to form large bipyramidal crystals identical to the *Charcot-Leyden crystals* ordinarily associated with eosinophilic inflammatory reactions (**Figure 35-2**, ×1,260). The refractile glassy blue structure, 25 by 5 µm in size, is composed of crystalline lysophospholipase that had oozed from basophilic and eosinophilic granules released by the disintegrating eosinophils. Surrounding this exotic splinter in **Figure 35-2** (starting at 6 o'clock) are "basophilic eosinophils" young and old, a myeloblast, a monoblast, and the wreckage of nucleolated cell—all basted with blue and pink granules. Apart from their granular chimerism, the dysplastic eosinophil precursors are exceptional for being anomalously positive for chloroacetate esterase.

Acute monocytic leukemia (AMoL) is characterized by high white counts, large ameboid leukemic cells, and marked elevations of plasma and urinary muramidase. AMoL occurs in 2 distinct forms. In the poorly differentiated subset (M5$_a$), the cells are very large and unequal in size and shape, and the voluminous basophilic cytoplasm (often containing clear vacuoles) is darkened peripherally, emphasizing a striking nuclear hof (**Figure 35-3**, ×2,000). The huge, variform, primitive, often folded or creased nuclei have reddish coralline chromatin containing ominously large nucleoli. In AMoL with partial differentiation (M5$_b$ variant), marrow and blood are inundated with a mixture of monoblasts, promonocytes, and young monocytes (**Figure 35-4**, ×2,000). The upper 2 cells in **Figure 35-4** are young monocytes equipped with lobular or folded spongiform nuclei and agranular gray-blue cytoplasm. Below them are 2 promonocytes with scant blue cytoplasm and twisted nuclei plus a nondescript rounded monoblast. Leukemic monocytes in M5 blood are sometimes lightly sprinkled with peroxidase-positive granules, and Auer rods are occasionally present. Differentiation from M2 and M4 variants and from microgranular APL can be certified by use of cytochemical stains. Monocyte-specific nonspecific esterase activity, using α-naphthyl butyrate as substrate and hexa-azotized pararosaniline as coupler, is the most specific cytochemical proof of AMoL. α-Naphthyl acetate and naphthol AS-D acetate are also reactive substrates for monocytes, but specificity must be validated by demonstrating inhibition by fluoride, a unique feature of monocyte esterases.

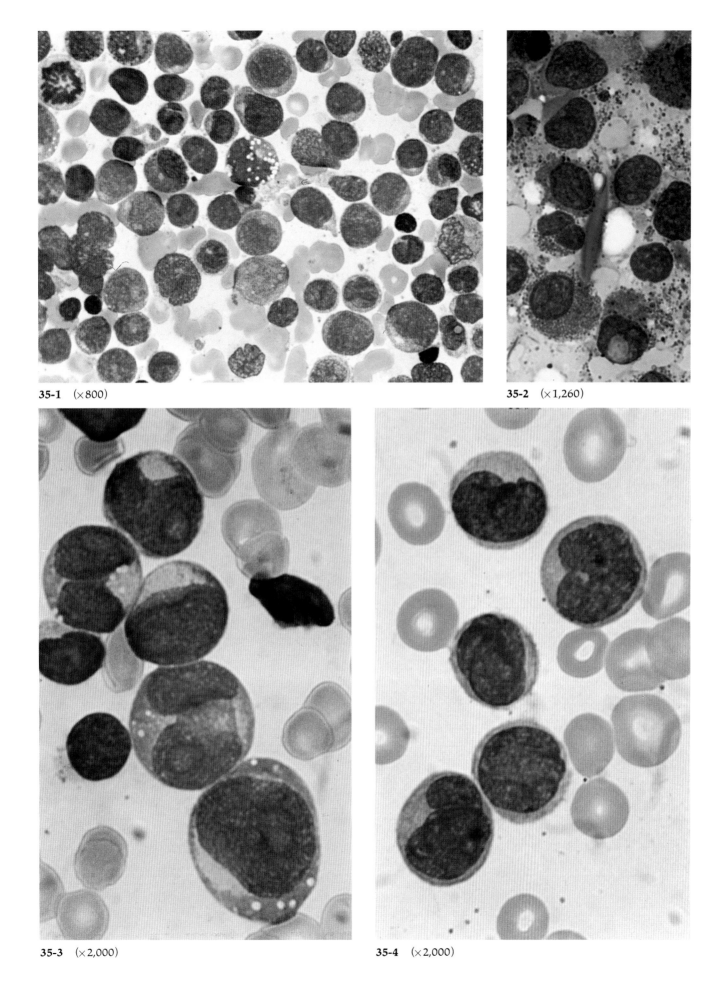

35-1 (×800)

35-2 (×1,260)

35-3 (×2,000)

35-4 (×2,000)

Figure 36. Erythroleukemia. Megakaryoblastic Leukemia.

Acute erythroleukemia (AEL), alias *DiGuglielmo's syndrome* or AML M6, accounts for only 4 to 6% of AMLs occurring de novo but contributes nearly 20% of leukemias secondary to alkylator therapy, irradiation, or overexposure to benzene. This high-echelon clonal disorder pursues a quirky chameleon course, with marrow patterns shifting unpredictably from exuberant erythroid hyperplasia to overt myeloblastic leukemia. Often emerging from a pre-existing myelodysplastic syndrome with erythroid predominance, erythroleukemia identifies itself in its early stages by spawning grotesque multinucleated erythroid monsters, such as the eye-poppers shown in **Figures 36-1** (×2,000) and **36-2** (×1,260). Marrow is richly cellular, occupied predominantly by colonies and sheets of erythroblasts, most of which have a megaloblastoid cast reminiscent of the moderately dysplastic morphology of refractory or hemolytic anemias. Erythroid hyperplasia is associated with assorted perversions in maturation-division, resulting in numerous dysplastic, megaloblastic, and lobulated nuclear forms. Karyorrhexis may be extensive. None of these changes is pathognomonic, and, as in Hodgkin's disease, a search must be made for the logos of erythroleukemia: multinucleated or polyploid erythroblasts (**Figure 36-1**) and the elusive but emblematic "gigantoblasts" (**Figure 36-2**). Hematologic parlance has no words for so massive a biologic mistake as the miscreation portrayed in **Figure 36-2** ensconced among its dysplastic progeny. In most cases of AEL, the vigorous but perverted proliferations are interrupted early by colonies of myeloblasts and by patchy myelofibrosis. Sooner or later the capricious excursions in cellularity and lineage eventuate in overgrowth by myeloblasts possessing M1 or M2 morphology, attesting to the pluripotential site of the clonal lesion. The erythroid nature of the DiGuglielmo phase of AEL usually is obvious by routine panoptic stains. In patients with numerous discolored proerythroblasts such as the curious polyploid cells in **Figure 36-1**, one of which has megakaryoblastoid "ears," detection of chunky PAS positivity and phenotyping with monoclonal antibodies to glycophorin A affirm erythroidhood. If the patient does not succumb to thrombocytopenic purpura, anemia, and infection secondary to marrow replacement, myeloblastic expansion quickly brings the course to a solemn conclusion.

Megakaryoblastic leukemia (acute myelofibrosis) is an unusual variant of acute myelogenous leukemia (AML M7), characterized by pancytopenia, initially-low blood blast levels, absence of hepatosplenomegaly, and ineffectual efforts to aspirate marrow ("dry taps"). Marrow is infiltrated early by sheets or clusters of dysplastic megakaryocytes; local leakage from these leukemic cells of *platelet-derived growth factor* and other fibroblast mitogens plus platelet factor 4 is responsible for the fibrotic webbing in which marrow cells are ensnared. Marrow biopsy reveals congeries of dysplastic megakaryoblasts, megakaryocytes, and megakaryocyte fragments. Most megakaryocytes are mononuclear, with pale blue hypogranular cytoplasm, knobby or earlike protrusions, and dark rounded nuclei with a single large nucleolus. Even when machine counts are ambivalent, blood morphology can provide a field of information (**Figure 36-3**, ×1,260). Shown here are seven dwarf mononuclear megakaryocytes, identifiable in several instances by their dappled pink cytoplasm, representing the pointillistic patterns of platelet territories. Megakaryocyte fragments in the company of nondescript fringed nuclei and giant platelets (some activated into a stellate conformation) are indisputable clues to diagnosis. The strange mononuclear forms lacking megakaryocyte cytoplasm somewhat resemble lymphoblasts except for their peculiar, puddled nuclear chromatin. These strange dwarf forms can also be difficult to distinguish from micromyeloblasts by routine Wright-Giemsa staining, although special stains reveal absence of sudanophilia and peroxidase activity. Identity of the anonymous blast cells and of their fragments is verified most readily by use of fluorescent monoclonal antibodies against platelet glycoproteins IIb-IIIa (CDw41), von Willebrand factor, and factor VIII. More laborious identification can be made by demonstrating platelet peroxidase activity in the nuclear envelope and endoplasmic reticulum by use of ultrastructural cytochemistry.

Megakaryoblastic leukemia is a fulminant disorder that moves swiftly from a myelofibrotic process to terminal megakaryoblastic leukemia; as in erythroleukemia, the denouement often involves acute transformation to an M1 or M2 version of AML. Blast transformation of Ph+ CML to a facsimile of acute megakaryocytic leukemia is relatively common; these 2 deadly processes can be distinguished by history, spleen size, and cytogenetics.

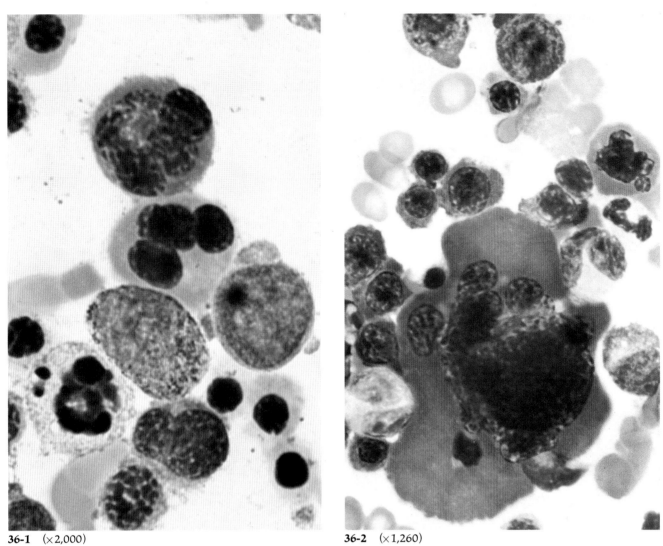

36-1 (×2,000)

36-2 (×1,260)

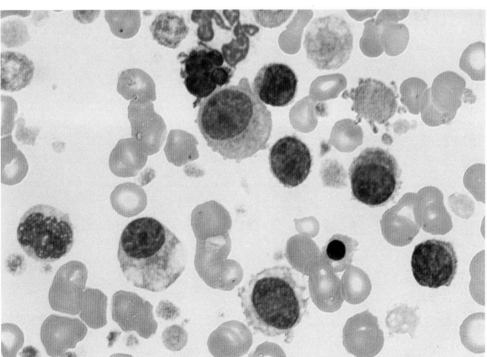

36-3 (×1,260)

Chronic Myeloproliferative Disorders

Figure 37. Chronic Myelogenous Leukemia: Chronic Phase and Accelerated Phase (Acute Transformation).

Chronic myelogenous leukemia (CML) is a clonal myeloproliferative disorder characterized by ceaseless overproduction of granulocytes and their precursors, most of which appear normal but are functionally somewhat defective. CML is remarkable for its programmed triphasic course consisting of an initial *chronic phase* of mounting granulocytosis, a transitional *accelerated phase*, and a murderous climax known as *blast crisis*. Diagnosis of chronic phase CML is quite obvious on low-power examination of blood smears (**Figure 37-1**, ×800), as all stages of normal myeloid differentiation are represented in rank order but display a symmetric shift toward immaturity. White counts at presentation are high, averaging nearly 200,000 cells/μl (range 20,000 to more than 1,000,000), and blood differential counts show a complete spectrum of differentiating forms, as though marrow had leaked into circulation. Several myeloproliferative signatures are visible in **Figure 37-1**: myelocytes and metamyelocytes are overrepresented (the 2 cells at top), denoting reiterative midstage divisions; basophils are ominously increased (right center); and platelets are swarming over the field, indicating inclusion of megakaryocyte precursors in the frenetic clone. That CML is a clonal disorder of the multipotential stem cell has been demonstrated by G6PD isozyme analysis, which indicates that the neoplastic founder clone encompasses neutrophils, eosinophils, basophils, erythroblasts, platelets, monocytes, B cells, and some T cells—hence the potential for any of these cell lines to participate in the explosive finale leading to blast crisis. Inspection of **Figure 37-1** leaves little reason for diagnostic equivocation. The sheer abundance of granulocytic forms is rather extreme for a leukemoid reaction to infection, and the triple hallmarks of sepsis (toxic granules, Döhle bodies, and neutrophil vacuolation) are absent. AML is out of contention, for there is no leukemic hiatus and no tyranny by myeloblasts in this full-spectrum populist pleomorphism. Thrombocythemia of this magnitude (platelet count was 3,000,000/μl) is almost never achieved during reactive thrombocytosis accompanying solid tumors, iron deficiency, or infection. The principal contestants are the other 3 chronic myeloproliferative syndromes: *idiopathic myelofibrosis, polycythemia vera,* and *idiopathic thrombocythemia*. Although they overlap in many clinical and laboratory features, none of these myeloproliferative disorders is ordinarily associated with granulocyte counts in excess of 50,000/μl. In perplexing cases having mixed or intermediate features, diagnostic reliance can be placed on chromosome analysis and cytochemical staining for *leukocyte alkaline phosphatase* (LAP). The cytogenetic cachet of CML is the *Philadelphia (Ph) chromosome*, a small but celebrated product of a 9;21 translocation, which fuses the *abl* oncogene of chromosome 9 to the broken end of the breakpoint cluster region *(bcr)* of chromosome 22. The resultant *bcr-abl* fusion gene transcript codes for a chimeric protein having remarkably robust growth factor activity that somehow accelerates myelopoiesis. Among the functional flaws affecting CML granulocytes is a diagnostic reduction in LAP. Normally, at least 20% of mature neutrophils show vigorous LAP activity, but in nearly all patients with uncomplicated chronic phase CML, enzyme activity in segmented neutrophils is absent or markedly diminished. LAP scores are generally normal or elevated in patients with granulocytosis accompanying polycythemia vera or idiopathic myelofibrosis, a useful distinction in segregating these kindred disorders.

Marrow biopsy or aspiration adds surprisingly little diagnostic information in CML. **Figure 37-2** (×800) reveals pronounced hypercellularity and exuberant myeloid proliferation, with a shift toward immaturity, to be expected in a patient with the blood picture shown in **Figure 37-1**. Myeloid heterogeneity distinguishes this chronic myeloproliferative pattern from the antisocial blast clusters of acute leukemia. Although erythroid elements are outnumbered (M : E ratio is about 20 : 1) and some erythroblasts are unavoidably pushed out into the bloodstream by the crush of myeloid proliferation, viable-looking erythroblasts can be seen milling around. The clear deep-blue cytoplasm of the several proerythroblasts at the lower left sets them off in this crowd of variably violaceous myeloid cells.

Figure 37-3 (×800) is a blood smear of the same patient portrayed in **Figures 37-1** and **37-2** as it looked 2½ years later at the outset of acute transformation. It is evident from this low-power view that granulocyte numbers have more than doubled, that platelets are much less numerous, and that the rank order of early myeloid precursors is reversed and skewed toward immaturity, with promyelocytes and young myelocytes dominating the scene. As only 2 or 3 myeloblasts are present (near center field), the patient could not be described as having entered blast crisis, but the adverse shift toward immature forms is ample forewarning of an impending "blast-off." Among the significant incidentals to this grim prospect are an orthochromatic erythroblast at left, a teardrop form signifying splenomegaly, the megakaryocyte fragment indicating infiltrative myelopathy, and the sinister basophil at upper left. Acute transformation can sometimes be stalled but never prevented from progressing to that most deadly of leukemic processes, blast crisis.

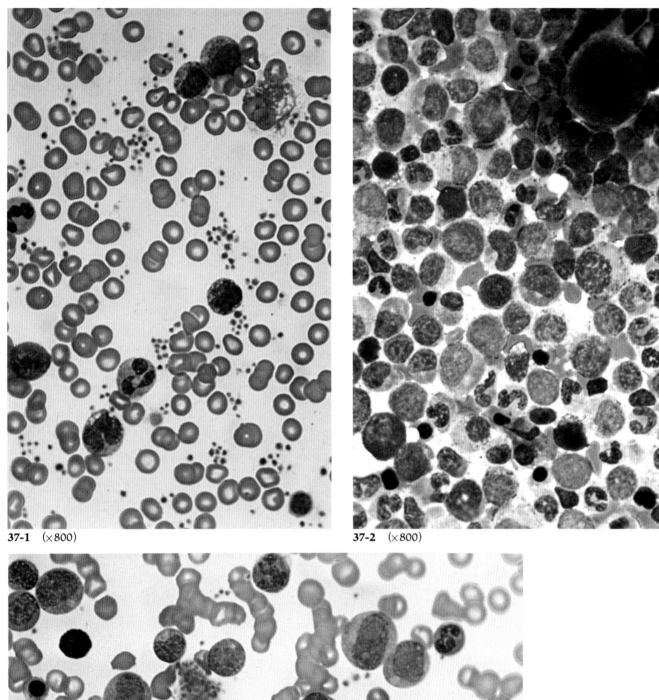

37-1 (×800)

37-2 (×800)

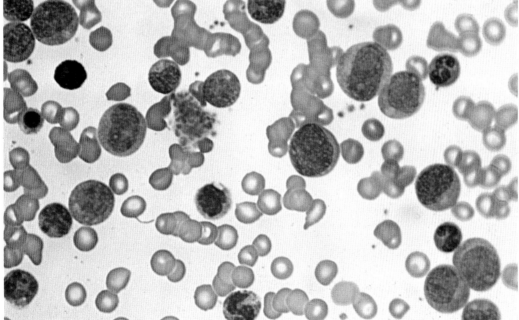

37-3 (×800)

Figure 38. Chronic Myelogenous Leukemia in Acute Transformation. Sea Blue Histiocyte. Pseudo-Gaucher Cells.

Blast crisis is a preordained sequel to chronic phase CML, coming on roughly 3 to 4 years after diagnosis, regardless of prior responsiveness to chemotherapy. Prophetic symptoms of the acute transformation prelude to blast crisis are inexplicable malaise and fever that may anticipate any change in blood counts. The grim beginning of this malign metamorphosis is soon evidenced by sudden emergence in blood of blasts and promyelocytes (**Figure 38-1**, ×800). As this accelerated phase takes hold, a burgeoning population of myeloblasts (center of figure) and dysplastic promyelocytes (largish cells at top and bottom) may so outnumber intermediate forms (myelocytes and metamyelocytes) that a leukemic hiatus is created, reminiscent of that in AML. Granulocyte levels may climb to prodigious heights, causing the blood to look milky as counts approach 1,000,000 cells/μl. Advent of acute transformation is often heralded by a surge in the number of those diviners of disaster, basophils, 2 of which are seen at the right in **Figure 38-1**. This field also includes a classic bilobed pseudo-Pelger cell at bottom center and shows a dearth of platelets, connoting collapse of normal hematopoiesis. Transformation to blast crisis results from malign evolution of subclones of stem cells bearing the fateful Ph chromosome, and during this accelerated phase additional chromosomal anomalies develop, the most common of which is a doubling of the Ph chromosome itself (+Ph). Clonal evolution ushers in an expansion of blast numbers so profound that the blood and marrow examined at this instant may closely mimic AML. Four criteria help differentiate myeloid blast crisis from AML. (1) Most CML patients in blast phase present with marked splenomegaly and a several-year history of ill health; most AML patients do not. (2) Basophil levels are nearly always elevated in CML and rise further during blast crisis; in AML basophilia is uncommon. (3) During blast crisis some intermediate myeloid forms persist, whereas in AML a leukemic hiatus (myeloblasts but no myelocytes) is usually striking. (4) The finding of 1 or more Ph chromosomes strongly favors blast crisis of CML, for in AML the t(9;22) translocation is rare (1%), is always singular, and usually results in an atypical fusion protein.

Escalation of blast and promyelocyte numbers during acute transformation characteristically is accompanied by deterioration in structure of these clonal progeny. Visible evidence of this is the finding of dysplastic (oversized) granules, in which basophilic and eosinophilic secondary granules are admixed or fused. Granular chimerism and leakage of granules into the neighborhood are seen occasionally in normal marrow, are common in chronic phase CML, and may become conspicuous during unfolding blast crisis, as demonstrated in **Figure 38-2** (×2,000). The trio of gaily decorated dysplastic promyelocytes surrounding the myeloblast at the center of this marrow field display a mixture of pink and black granules, some of which are being shed into the surroundings. The 3 myeloblasts at the lower left display anisoblastosis characteristic of blast crisis. The 2 smaller M1 blasts are vacuolated, as is often true of leukemic cells, and the large cell with cytoplasmic granules and brainy-looking chromatin was arrested at a more mature (M2) stage of differentiation. Inclusion within the clone of myeloblasts (young and old) plus promyelocytes justifies counting both progenitor stages in establishing a diagnosis of leukemia.

The tropical azure and sparkling cytoplasmic highlights flaunted by the cell in **Figure 38-3** (×1,260) attest to the aptness of the term *sea blue histiocyte*. Enormous (50 to 60 μm across) lipid-stuffed marrow macrophages, whose curdled contents are stained blue-green by Wright-Giemsa, sea blue histiocytes, however charming their color, are simply ponderous victims of their own gulosity. Macrophages covet membrane lipids, including the indigestible ceroids responsible for their travelogue tints. Hence these pastel giants, to their own distress, accumulate in hematologic disorders featuring massively increased local blood cell destruction, of which CML and thalassemia are exemplary. Sea blue histiocytes also appear in Niemann-Pick disease, in which the daily load of ceroids such as sphingomyelin is normal but macrophages are deficient in sphingomyelinase. Blue-green granulation on Wright-Giemsa staining is not specific for ceroids; it is also produced by hemosiderin, malaria pigment, and melanin. Sea blue histiocytes of CML differ subtly in displaying superficial flecks of purple, the half-digested remains of deceased granulocytes and platelets.

The *pseudo-Gaucher cells* (**Figure 38-4**, ×600) encountered in the marrow in CML and other chronic proliferative states, including multiple myeloma, are indistinguishable by light microscopy from the cells of Gaucher's disease. The Gaucher-like cells of proliferative disorders are not caused by deficiency of glucocerebrosidase (as in the eponymic original): the enzyme is not lacking, it is overwhelmed. **Figure 38-4** reveals 4 Gaucherlike cells nested among marrow cells of a patient with multiple myeloma. The cytoplasm of these storage macrophages (1 of which is binucleate) has the appearance of combed or balled yarn; the illusion is created by pale strands of cerebroside inclusions set off against the pale blue macrophage cytoplasm. In CML it is not unusual to encounter several picturesque kinds of lipid storage cells.

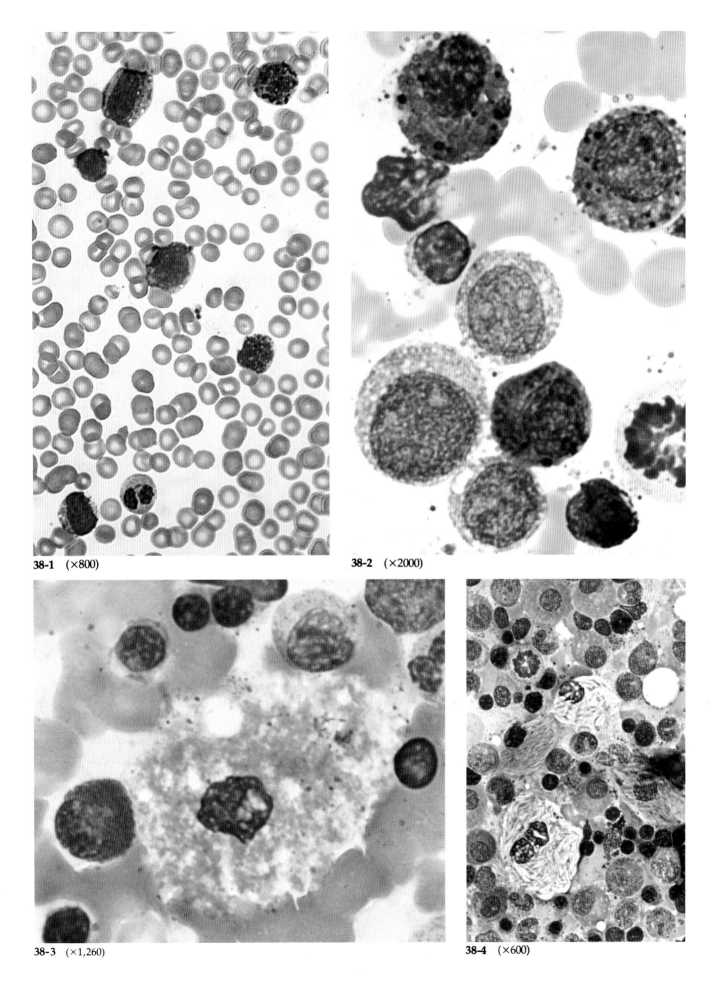

38-1 (×800)

38-2 (×2000)

38-3 (×1,260)

38-4 (×600)

Figure 39. Blast Phase of Chronic Myelogenous Leukemia

The programmed finale to chronic phase CML is a sudden acceleration in the pace of proliferation known as the *blast phase* or *blast crisis*. This biological eruption represents an ordained, uncontrollable impulse on the part of the neoplastic stem cell to select for mass production a single line of committed blast forms, recruited from its extended clonal family. The extraordinary diversity of cell lines generated during the blast phase in various patients with CML bears out isozyme and cell marker evidence that the founder cell is grandparent to all myeloid lines of CFU-GEMM as well as of some lymphoid lines. Most patients (65%) experience myeloid blast crisis (**Figure 39-1**), a large minority (20%) enter a lymphoid crisis (**Figure 39-2**), and the remainder of these blastic outbursts (about 5% each) feature DiGuglielmo type erythroblasts, monoblasts (**Figure 39-3**), or megakaryoblasts (**Figure 39-4**). The variegate expression of blast crisis and the occurrence, in many instances, of mixed-blast crises or overgrowth of blast forms having biphenotypic or multilineage markers places the initial leukemogenic lesion at the most sovereign hematopoietic stem cell level. In classic AML the mutant cells are committed CFUs from the start, and the disease presents in "blast crisis," all the multiple steps of leukemogenesis having occurred simultaneously. In CML these steps evolve sequentially, and only after a long "pre-leukemic" chronic phase does 1 of the committed clonal cell lines "blast off" into an acute leukemia.

Metamorphosis into blast phase sometimes occurs explosively ("true" blast crisis), but more often it is ushered in by an unstable period lasting several months marked by deteriorating health, recurrence of splenomegaly, and gradual escape of white counts from therapeutic control. Other dark premonitions heralding blastic change include worsening anemia and thrombocytopenia and rising basophilia. Any adverse change in clinical or hematologic aspects of chronic phase should forewarn of incipient acceleration. Common cytogenetic signs of evolution to blast phase include duplication of the pre-existing Ph chromosome or addition of new nonrandom anomalies, including variant Ph translocations, trisomy 8, trisomy 19, and replacement of normal chromosome 17 by an isochromosome, i(17q). An unusual, often baffling, early form of acute transformation is emergence of *extramedullary myeloblastomas (granulocytic sarcomas)* in bone, lymph nodes, skin, or breast, often preceding blood or marrow evidence of blast phase.

In approximately two-thirds of patients, blast phase represents a myeloid detonation, in which malignant myeloblasts overrun the marrow and spill into the bloodstream (**Figure 39-1**, ×1,260). Usually undifferentiated M1 type myeloblasts predominate, as shown in this figure, and display considerable heterogeneity in size and shape similar to that of AML. Nucleoli are large and irregular, and a few red granules may be visible, but (unlike AML) Auer rods are almost never encountered. Note the basophil, the pelgeroid neutrophil, and the ultimate in nuclear : cytoplasmic dyssynchrony—a body of cytoplasm *sans* nucleus. When, as in this instance, the myeloblasts are so poorly differentiated that cytochemical markers (peroxidase, Sudan black B, specific esterase) give negative or equivocal results, *immunophenotyping* using monoclonal antibodies may often (but not always) settle the issue. Markers indicating myeloidhood include antibodies to the MY7 (CD13) and MY9 (CD33) antigens.

During lymphoid blast crisis (**Figure 39-2**, ×1,260) the dominant cells have characteristic lymphoblast morphology and in most cases are phenotypically and visibly similar to the pre B cells of common ALL. The lymphoid cells are positive for terminal deoxynucleotidyl transferase (TdT) and HLA-DR, express the *CALL antigen* (CALLA), contain cytoplasmic Ig μ chains, and display clonal immunoglobulin gene rearrangements. Lymphoblasts in lymphoid blast crisis are unmistakable in their morphologic lineaments, showing typical heavily smudged chromatin and oblong or angular (often triangular) nuclei thinly cloaked in deep clear-blue agranular cytoplasm. The clonal population usually includes numerous small, friendly looking lymphocytes as an added visual aid. In exceptional cases blast cells bear the T cell phenotype and show clonal rearrangement of T cell antigen receptor genes. More than half of patients with lymphoid blast crisis respond well, if transiently, to "anti-ALL" therapy. Some crises present as mixtures of lymphoid and myeloid blast forms or may shift their lineage from predominantly lymphoid to myeloid; such malignant mixtures can be stained with selective monoclonal antibodies and then separated by use of *fluorescence-activated cell sorters*.

Every member of the FAB 7 clan can crop up as the dominant cell during blast crisis, including APL cells and, as shown in **Figure 39-3** (×1,260), monoblasts resembling those of AMoL. This mixture of monoblasts and promonocytes parades every contortion of which a bulbous nucleus is capable, plus a few French modifications. No special stains are demanded, but these ameboid cells can be certified by demonstrating nonspecific esterase positivity and the monocyte phenotype of CD13, CD14, and CD11. Note the 2 basophils as a reminder of the myeloproliferative origins of these blasts.

Megakaryoblastic crisis in CML (**Figure 39-4**, ×1,260) affords an opportunity to review the manifold guises of which megakaryoblast fragments are capable. Megakaryoblast fragments, or *micromegakaryocytes*, the only forms small enough to enter the bloodstream, are usually mononuclear or bilobed and may or may not possess the telltale platelet-dappled cytoplasm which gives away the cell at bottom right. Micromegakaryocytes can be very difficult to identify when stripped of cytoplasm (as with the 2 nuclear blobs toward the center), and in this scene the numerous large, even giant, platelet forms are strong leads to diagnosis. Micromegakaryocytes having scant blue cytoplasm and large dense nuclei with small nucleoli often resemble lymphoblasts. Cytochemical studies may reveal punctate positivity for nonspecific esterase and for PAS and strong, diffuse reactivity to specific esterase staining. More decisive identification can be achieved by using monoclonal antibodies to platelet glycoproteins Ib, IIb-IIIa, von Willebrand factor, and factor VIII, or by the arduous demonstration by electron microscopy (EM) of platelet peroxidase reactivity.

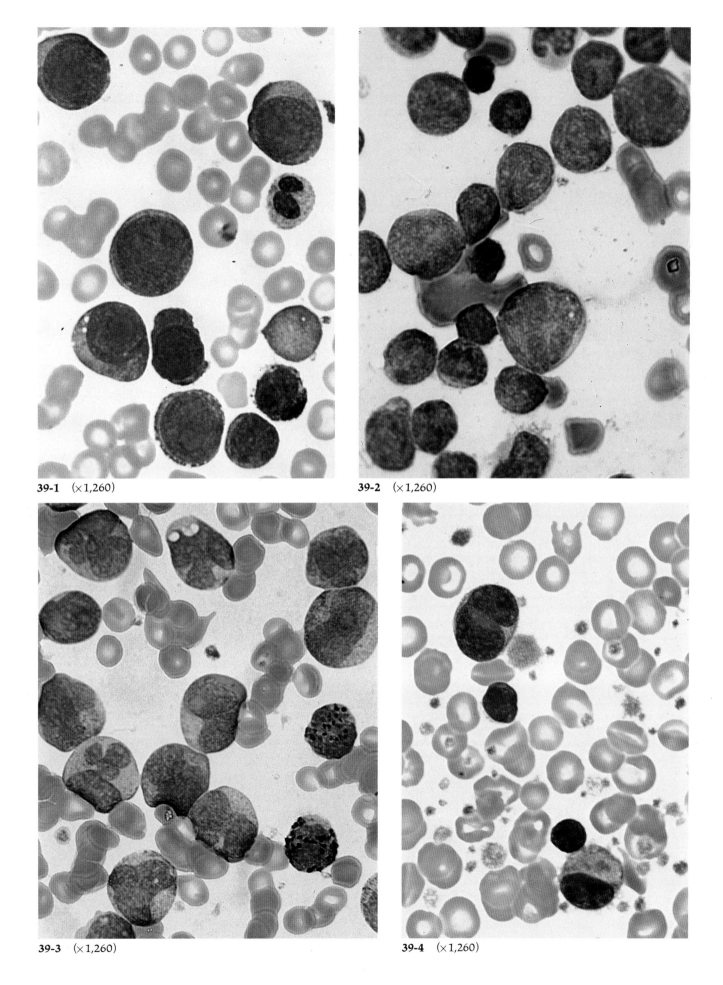

39-1 (×1,260)

39-2 (×1,260)

39-3 (×1,260)

39-4 (×1,260)

Figure 40. Idiopathic Myelofibrosis

Idiopathic myelofibrosis is a peculiar and insidious form of chronic myeloproliferative disease dominated by the combined consequences of infiltrative myelopathy and splenomegaly secondary to extramedullary hematopoiesis *(myeloid metaplasia)*. The complex morphologic findings in blood are teardrop deformities, anomalous emergence of nucleated red cells and early myeloid forms, and giant platelets often accompanied by megakaryocyte fragments (**Figures 40-1 through 40-3**). **Figure 40-1** ($\times1,260$) shows a normal neutrophil in the presence of an orthochromatic erythroblast and a young myeloblast. The questions raised by this troublesome trio are answered by the surrounding collection of teardrop deformities. Nearly one-fourth of the red cells have tails, a frequency of teardrop deformation found only in thalassemia major (which this patently is not) and myelofibrosis. A lower-power view (**Figure 40-2,** $\times800$) in a patient with a white cell count exceeding 100,000 per μl introduces the possibility of CML because of the association of 3 myelocytes (aligned vertically at the upper center) in the company of a band form, 2 neutrophils, an eosinophil, and the always-suspect basophil (at 3 o'clock), plus a pelgeroid cell (bottom left). The sheer numbers of teardrop-shaped red cells in this field steer one toward myelofibrosis, but the distinction from CML in patients with high granulocyte levels, medullary fibrosis, and extramedullary (splenic) hematopoiesis is difficult. In this case, 2 findings served to exclude CML from the differential diagnosis between these sister syndromes: the LAP score was high, and chromosomal analysis failed to unearth a Ph chromosome.

Myelofibrosis is an acquired clonal disorder originating in a single pluripotential stem cell. The EP-independent erythroblasts that colonize the spleen, the superfluous myeloid cells of all ages that roam the circulation, and the megakaryocyte populations that flourish in marrow and disrupt its architecture are all products of this single mutant but versatile clone. *Dysmegakaryocytopoiesis* with overproduction of defective platelets is the central pathogenic feature. Clusters of dysplastic megakaryocytes collect and proliferate in vascular sinuses of both marrow and spleen, discharging into the environment high levels of the potent fibroblast mitogen, platelet-derived growth factor (PDGF). With time, nests of dysplastic megakaryocytes become imprisoned (along with other marrow elements) by a fibrotic webbing induced by their own sickly secretions. The resulting dense reticulin fibrosis laid down by nonclonal fibroblasts displaces marrow parenchyma and is responsible for promoting emigration of hematopoietic stem cells to the spleen and other sites. Continued seepage of PDGF and platelet factor 4 from the dysplastic, moribund megakaryocytes causes a collagen gridlock in marrow, which is responsible for dry taps on attempted needle aspiration. Fibrosis also scars and deforms the exits of the marrow : blood barrier, accounting for the escape of immature marrow cells, including fragments of megakaryocytes themselves, into circulation. **Figure 40-3** ($\times1,260$) displays an apparent binucleate cell, which in reality is a dysplastic *megakaryocyte fragment*. Its identity is evident from the characteristic deep purple nuclear masses, the peppered pattern of the cytoplasm, and several earlike cytoplasmic flaps. The neighboring myelophthisic array (proceeding clockwise) of a band form, a metamyelocyte, a late promyelocyte, and an early band complete the myelofibrotic pastiche.

Figure 40-4 ($\times800$) presents a blood smear from a patient with both hemoglobin S–thalassemia and idiopathic myelofibrosis. Removal of the spleen erased the telltale teardrop deformities characteristic of both thalassemia and myelofibrosis but enabled a farrago of leukoerythroblastic forms to flood into circulation. At lower center is a mononuclear *dwarf megakaryocyte*, adorned with tags and tassels of cytoplasm. When very abundant these mononuclear forms with their dark nondescript nuclei can be puzzling, final identification requiring use of special markers such as monoclonal anti-platelet antibodies or ultrastructural cytochemistry with the platelet peroxidase reaction. In this instance the picturesque leukoerythroblastic setting is sufficient evidence for a myeloproliferative disorder. Proceeding clockwise from the top are: a basophil, a late promyelocyte, a promyelocyte paired with a late myelocyte, the dwarf megakaryocyte, a late myelocyte leaning on a neutrophil, and (at 10 o'clock) a dysplastic myeloblast. A late erythroblast is at the center of this circle of cells. A thalassemia gene is responsible for the microcytosis and hypochromia, thin wafer forms and folded cells being characteristic of thalassemia after splenectomy.

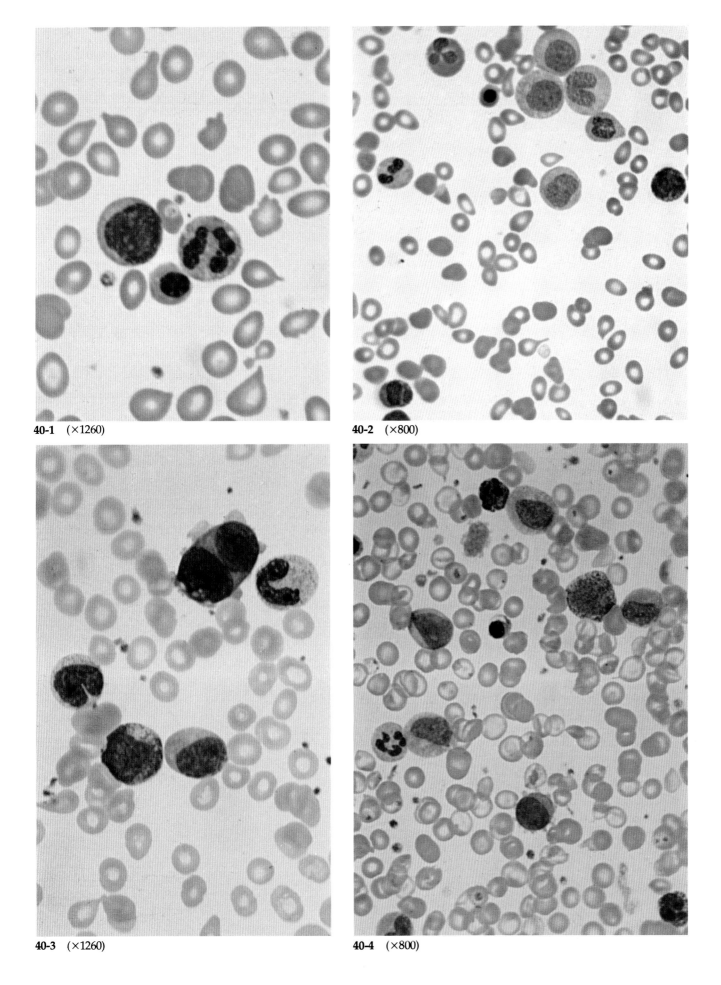

40-1 (×1260)

40-2 (×800)

40-3 (×1260)

40-4 (×800)

Acute Lymphatic Leukemia

Figure 41. Acute Lymphatic Leukemia: Blood Findings

Acute lymphatic leukemia (acute lymphoblastic leukemia; ALL) is a clonal malignancy arising from committed lymphopoietic stem cells of marrow. Initially malignant lymphoblasts remain and accumulate in marrow, crowding out the more civil hematopoietic elements, but eventually tumor cells emerge and flood the bloodstream (**Figures 41-1** through **41-3**).

Three morphologic subsets of ALL have been defined by criteria set forth by French-American-British (FAB) grandees. In the L1 subtype found predominantly in children 10 years of age or younger, lymphoblasts are uniformly small, nuclei are round and regular, and the sparse cytoplasm is midnight blue. **Figure 41-2** ($\times 2,000$) illustrates the monotonous conformity of a cluster of L1 lymphoblasts. (Clusters always connote cancer.) Their plump round or faintly scalloped nuclei occupy most of the cell volume, creating a nuclear : cytoplasmic ratio far in excess of $3:1$. Nuclear chromatin is blue-purple and is distinctly if irregularly granulated, lacking the vitreous smoothness and violaceous hue of myeloblast nuclei. The nuclear membrane is more distinct than that of myeloblasts, being thick and interrupted rather than thin and continuous. Nucleoli in L1 lymphoblasts are small and infrequent; many blasts lack discernible nucleoli, and those present are vaguely formed and smudged.

In adults and older children, ALL blast morphology is chiefly of the L2 sort (**Figure 41-1**, $\times 1,260$). L2 lymphoblasts are larger and more variable in size and shape than L1 blasts. Cytoplasm is abundant in some cells but sparse in most and has medium to deep blue margins. The rounded nuclei are often irregular, many show blunt folds or twists, and some are smoothly clefted. Many blasts contain bold nucleoli, 1 or 2 per cell, with circular craterlike contours accentuated by rims of aggregated chromatin. Normally lymphoblasts are inquisitive creatures, employing a posterior extension known as the *uropod* for sensing suspect surfaces. ALL blasts of all types may extend their sensory devices, as exemplified by the cell at lower left. When lymphoblasts in the uropod mode are numerous, the leukemia may be dubbed the *hand-mirror variant* of ALL, a label lacking prognostic significance. More germane to outcome is the relative proportions of blasts having L1 or L2 characteristics, for in most patients with ALL who are older than 8 or 10 years, blood and marrow contain mixtures of the 2. L2 morphology predicts poor response to chemotherapeutic induction, and the presence of as few as 10% L2 cells diminishes prospects for incident-free remission. For prognostic purposes, presence of more than 90% L1 blasts (**Figure 41-2**), as is characteristic of "childhood ALL" occurring in the 2- to 7-year age group, is strongly predictive of sustained remission on appropriate therapy and a good (50%) chance of chemical cure. Patients (most of them adolescents and adults) in whom over half of lymphoblasts have large irregular nuclei and prominent nucleoli, as in **Figure 41-3** ($\times 2,000$), have a far less sunny outlook and more complex clonal lesions. In patients with intermediate blast mixtures (L1/L2 ALL and L2/L1 ALL), longterm event-free remission rates range from 10 to 30%, the 10-year survival rate being strongly subverted by increasing age.

Over 80% of ALLs represent clonal arrest of B cell lymphoblasts early in their maturation. Most ALL lymphoblasts express the specific B cell lineage marker CD19, the less specific CALLA (or CD10) and HLA-DR (Ia) antigens, and the mitogenic nuclear enzyme TdT. Hence, the phenotypic profile for the common early (pre-pre B) B cell ALLs is CD19+, CD10+, Ia+, and TdT+. This prevalent CALLA+ subset can be distinguished from the less common but more mature *pre B ALL* by presence in the latter of cytoplasmic µ chains, denoting early immunoglobulin synthesis. B cell progenitors are unique in undergoing clonal *immunoglobulin gene rearrangements* during ontogeny. In B cell ALL, these gene movements are halted early in development, resulting in clonal "immortalization" of incomplete rearrangements detectable by DNA probe analysis.

Nearly 20% of ALLs result from a block in thymocyte stages of T cell differentiation. Leukemic T cells may be indistinguishable morphologically from the common type B cell ALL, and those formed early in T cell differentiation are also TdT+; however, ALL blasts with convoluted or floral nuclear patterns almost always can be certified by marker studies as T cells. T cell ALL lymphoblasts are marked distinctively by the early thymic antigen CD7 (Leu9) and the pan-T markers CD3 and CD5. Most T cell ALLs express clonal rearrangements of the *T cell antigen receptors* (TcRs), which are demonstrable by restriction fragment analysis. T cell ALL is characterized by rapid progression, male predominance, high numbers of circulating blasts, meningeal involvement, and mediastinal or thymic adenopathy. Apart from phenotyping by use of fluorescent antibodies to TdT, CALLA, Ia, and surface or cytoplasmic immunoglobulins, the most useful cytochemical markers for profiling ALL blasts are the *PAS* and *acid phosphatase reactions*. In at least 70% of cases, ALL blasts display heavy red granular or chunky "block" patterns of PAS staining. Focal punctate or unipolar paranuclear staining reactions for acid phosphatase usually correlate well with proof of "T-ness" by cell marker and gene rearrangement data. Neither PAS nor focal acid phosphatase patterns are specific for ALL, and a full panel of markers or gene rearrangement studies may be required for diagnosis. In a small subset of ALL, lymphoblasts are trapped so early in differentiation that they express only the HLA-DR antigen and are termed *null cells*. Null cell ALL, which occurs largely in infants and older adults, appears to result from ineffective ("sterile") H chain rearrangements and is quite refractory to chemotherapy.

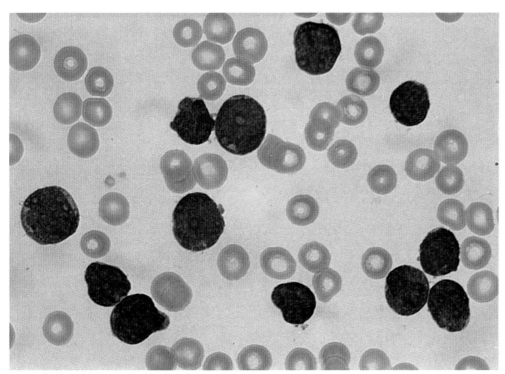

41-1 （×1,260）

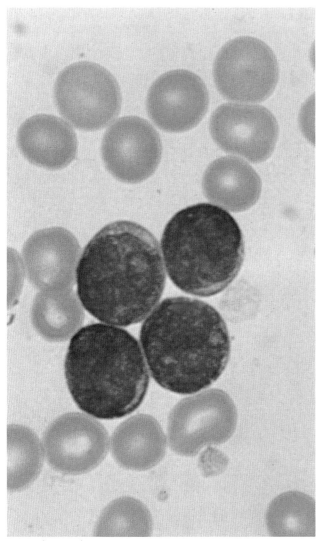

41-2 （×2,000）

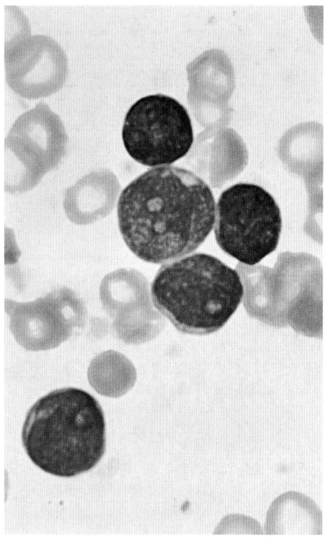

41-3 （×2,000）

Figure 42. Marrow in Acute Lymphatic Leukemia

Marrow replacement occurs at the outset in ALL. Unlike AML, invasion by leukemic blasts is unheralded by pre-leukemic phenomena, and there is nothing hesitant or constrained about the tumor cell irruption. Patients suffering from AML commonly present with "only" 30 to 40% blasts, but in ALL marrow space is crammed with lymphoblasts by the time of diagnosis (**Figure 42-1**, ×800). In this crowded battleground, hordes of lymphoblasts swarm over the terrain, leaving only a pair of myeloid cells and one embattled erythroblast (right-center). Near-total ablation of hematopoietic elements by lymphoblasts is responsible for the early anemia and thrombocytopenic purpura characteristic of ALL. Clinical manifestations and cytopenias reflect damage done to marrow, regardless of blast numbers in the blood. In both children and adults, about one-third of ALL patients have white counts below 5,000 cells/μl. Another third have counts in the normal range, and in the remainder white counts are elevated, exceeding 100,000 cells/μl in 15% of patients. When the total white count is below 5,000 cells/μl, leukemic blasts may be hard to find in blood; hence, as in oligoblastic AML, diagnosis in nearly half of ALL victims depends on marrow examination, where the lymphoblastic nature of the massive infiltrations is generally obvious.

Approximately 90% of ALLs afflict children, this leukemia accounting for one-fourth of all malignancies occurring before age 15. L1 morphology and good prospects of chemocurability typify childhood ALL, but during late adolescence and adulthood the L1 : L2 ratio inexorably swings toward the less favorable L2 disease (L1 : L2 ratio of 1 : 2). **Figures 42-1** and **42-2** (×2,000) are exemplary of lymphoblast populations found in adult-onset ALL. About two-thirds of the lymphoid blasts are variably large, some being twice the size of L1 lymphoblasts. Blast forms are pleomorphic and often display nuclear dents, clefts, or blunt lobules, and many have 1 or 2 small but stark nucleoli. The remainder of cells in both figures are small, dark, round, nondescript forms virtually devoid of cytoplasm—typical of L1 blasts. As noted in **Figure 41**, fewer than 20% of ALLs are T cell proliferations, most being of B cell lineage and possessing the marginally differentiated early pre B (pre-pre B) phenotype characteristic of childhood ALL. About 20% of ALLs express a pre B cell phenotype, with cytoplasmic immunoglobulin (cIg). Fewer than 3% of ALL cases flaunt the full phenotype of mature B cells, including L3 morphology and presence of surface (membrane) immunoglobulin (sIg). Although clonal chromosomal abnormalities are discoverable in over 90% of patients with ALL, only certain structural or numerical aberrations have clinical impact. Tumor cells in about 30% of childhood and 10% of adult cases are hyperdiploid (modal number, 47 to 60 chromosomes); hyperdiploidy with more than 50 chromosomes is a highly favorable prognostic indicator. Conversely, about one-third of adult and one-fifth of childhood ALLs are associated with 1 of 3 reciprocal translocations bearing a strongly adverse influence on outcome: t(4;11), t(8;14), and a 9;22 translocation grossly resembling that responsible for the Ph chromosome. The t(8;14) translocation, known as the *Burkitt's rearrangement*, is characteristic of *Burkitt's lymphoma* and of the L3 type of ALL.

The L3 variant of ALL is characterized by high blood blast levels, prominent extramedullary infiltrative masses, and a rapid downhill course refractory to chemotherapy. As illustrated in **Figure 42-3** (×1,260), L3 blasts recovered from marrow are quite large and have pleomorphic round or oblong nuclei with granular or slightly curdled violet chromatin, in which 1 to 5 nucleoli are embedded. The eccentric, capacious cytoplasm, which is variably basophilic, particularly along the margins, is laden with fatty inclusions that in Wright-Giemsa preparations appear as clear vacuoles. Note that this picturesque cluster of vacuolated blasts is surrounded by nonclonal myeloid elements, including band forms (top left) and 3 promyelocytes plus a myeloblast (near the bottom). L3 lymphoblasts are errant but mature sIg⁺ B cell blasts that have lost their cIg, CALLA, and TdT components. L3 ALL possesses an explosive replicative potential analogous to that of the fast-growing tumors of Burkitt's lymphoma, and in rare instances this high-grade solid tumor presents with leukemic blood involvement. In both the leukemia and lymphoma, clonal proliferation is ignited during fusion of the amputated terminal limb of the long arm of chromosome 8 (8q), which contains the *c-myc* oncogene, to the unstable immunoglobulin gene region on band 14q32. This juxtaposes *c-myc* genes and the transcriptionally tempestuous heavy chain gene region of B cells, which drives expression of *c-myc* to high levels and predisposes this oncogene to mutation. Exactly how fusion of *c-myc* to *Burkitt's band* triggers this specific and deadly variant of ALL is not known.

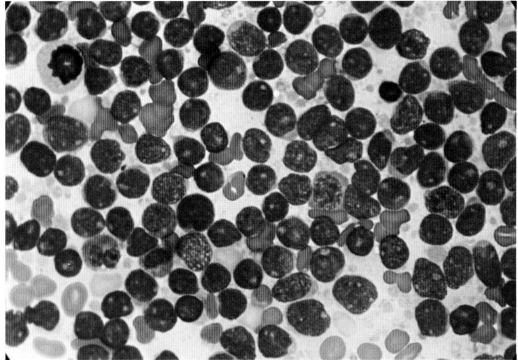

42-1　(×800)

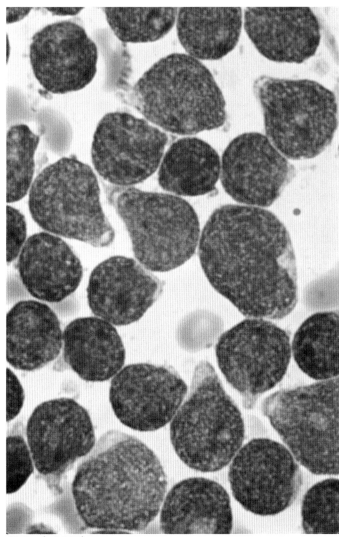

42-2　(×2,000)

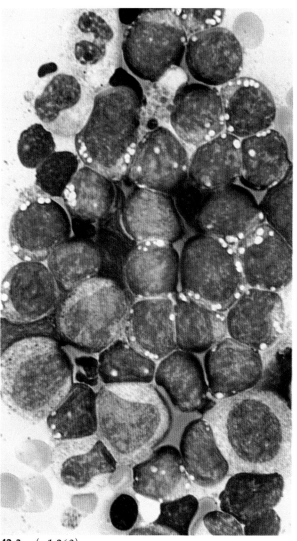

42-3　(×1,260)

Chronic Lymphatic Leukemia and Related Disorders

Figure 43. Chronic Lymphatic Leukemia

Chronic lymphatic leukemia (chronic lymphocytic leukemia, CLL) is the most chronic, most benign, and most age-dependent of hematopoietic neoplasms. Among other "mosts," it is most easily recognized on blood smears by the myriads of mature lymphocytes (**Figure 43-1**, ×800). Normally blood lymphocytes do not exceed about 4,000 cells/μl, and a provisional diagnosis of CLL should be made in any adult whose lymphocyte levels are persistently above 5,000/μl. During the early years of CLL the malignant population of lymphocytes appears homogeneous and harmless. On average, however, the tumor cells are slightly enlarged and some may burst during preparation of blood films, particularly when spread on slides, betraying their skeletal frailty. Presence of numerous *smudge cells,* such as those in **Figure 43-1**, is sufficiently suggestive of leukemia to warrant notation in the differential report. Chromatin in most cells is heavily clumped in a normal wadded pattern, but in a minority of lymphocytes the chromatin may appear excessive and chunky, and occasionally half-concealed small nucleoli may be seen peeking through. CLL is a languid lymphoproliferative disorder, but in its unhurried course lymphocyte numbers inexorably mount (unless reined back by chemotherapy or radiation) to very high levels, sometimes exceeding 1,000,000 cells/μl. As counts rise, cells accumulate in all tissues to which lymphocytes have access, and lymphadenopathy and splenomegaly occur early. In patients with more aggressive disease, the mutant lymphocytes become increasingly pleomorphic. Cells with scant cytoplasm may exhibit deeply cleaved or cracked nuclei and are sometimes known as *Rieder cells.* **Figure 43-3** (×1,260) shows a group of slightly enlarged CLL lymphocytes displaying various cleavage patterns. Lymphocytes with split (cleaved, cloven, cleft) or bisected nuclei are found abundantly in CLL and occur in smaller numbers in the blood of normal individuals exposed to excessive ionizing radiation or cytotoxic drugs. The fevered grammar of hematologists has generated many earthy terms for this most benign form of nuclear fission: among these are cracked, fissured, and buttock patterns.

Immunohemolytic anemia (IHA) occurs as an unpredictable complication in about 10% of patients with B cell CLL (B-CLL). The hemolytic interlude is nearly always mediated by warm-active IgG autoantibodies of low avidity and unknown objective. CLL is the most common pathologic process predisposing to *Coombs-positive hemolytic anemia,* creating a morphologic amalgam combining microspherocytic and polychromatophilic red cells with throngs of small lymphocytes and smudge cells (**Figure 42-2,** ×800). Hemolysis seldom strikes with the ferocity sometimes seen in idiopathic or drug-induced cases of IHA, but, as intimated by the pronounced spherocytosis and presence of a nucleated red cell, anemia can be sufficiently severe to require transfusional support. Blood findings reveal all of the trappings of hemolytic anemia (reticulocytosis, hyperbilirubinemia, exhaustion of haptoglobin, and erythroid hyperplasia) superimposed on the lymphoproliferative scenery. Note in **Figure 43-2** the ominous absence of platelets, suggesting either that the acute immune process also attacks platelets or that normal thrombopoiesis has been shut down by marrow infiltration. The orthochromatic erythroblast with the shamrock-shaped nucleus is preparing to expel its pyknotic chromatin. This is normal karyorrhexis but is sometimes misinterpreted as a dysplastic feature. IHA complicating CLL is managed in the same manner as other immunohemolytic anemias, until the process vanishes as mysteriously as it commenced.

Early in CLL, leukemic lymphocytes form nodular enclaves that simulate well-differentiated lymphocytic lymphoma, but, as infiltration spreads out and becomes confluent, normal hematopoietic elements are displaced, leading to deepening anemia, thrombocytopenia, and neutropenia. In **Figure 43-4** (×1,260) all but a few residents have been evicted from marrow space by the crush of mutant lymphocytes. Many of these lymphocytes appear slightly large, chromatin clumping is coarse and overly defined, and some cells have dented or folded nuclei. These features are subtle signs that the infiltrators are growing hostile and that normal hematopoietic cells are approaching extinction. The 2 outnumbered basophilic erythroblasts at lower right can be distinguished from the swarming lymphocytes by their darker (purpler) chromatin and more opaque cytoplasm. Usually when marrow is this crammed with CLL cells and either hemoglobin or platelet levels have declined substantially (clinical stage IV), prospects for survival beyond 2 years are small. CLL is second only to human immunodeficiency virus (HIV) infection as a cause of acquired immunodeficiency syndrome, and infection is the principal cause of death. This slow-paced malignancy also subjects patients to risk from secondary, more impetuous, malignant processes. Among these are poorly differentiated malign lymphomas *(Richter's syndrome)* and transformation to a more aggressive process, prolymphocytic leukemia.

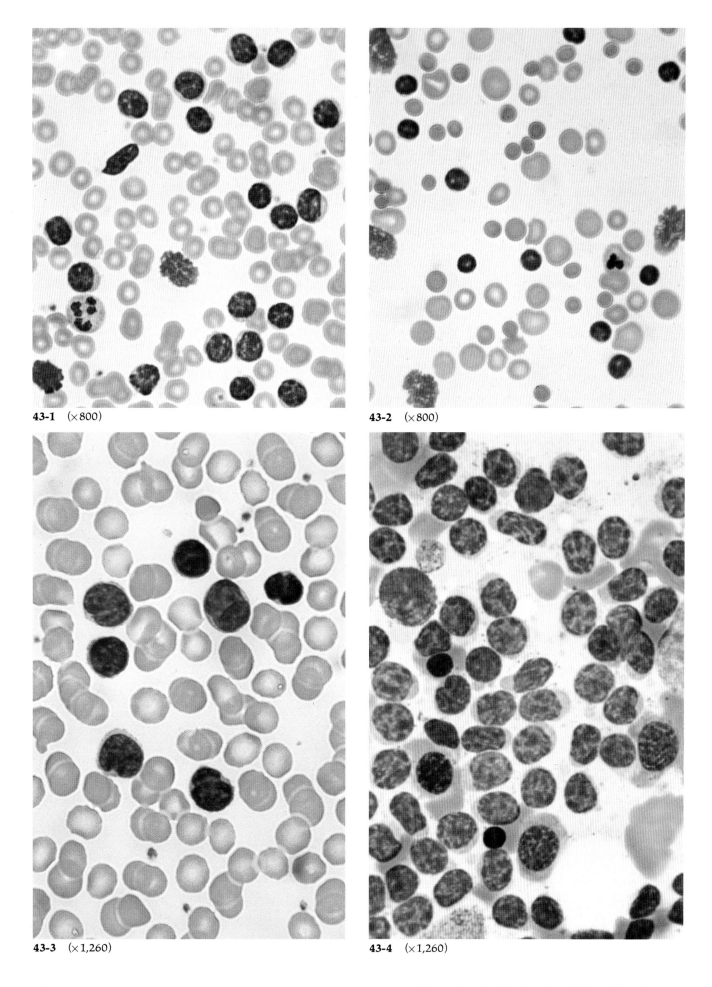

43-1 (×800)

43-2 (×800)

43-3 (×1,260)

43-4 (×1,260)

Figure 44. T Cell Chronic Lymphatic Leukemia. Prolymphocytic Leukemia. HTLV-I Infection. Lymphoma Cell Leukemia.

A minority of CLL cases are chronic T cell neoplasms. These are divisible into a rare T4 phenotype (T4-CLL) characterized by small cell morphology, marked lymphocytosis, and rapid progression; and T8 variants (T8-CLL) with NK morphology (**Figure 44-1**, ×2,000), low white counts, and an indolent course. T8-CLL comprises proliferations of *cytotoxic T cells* that have undergone clonal rearrangements of the T cell antigen receptor (TcR), as well as look-alike disorders having the phenotypic emblems of NK-hood. Although their genealogies are obscured by phenotypic infidelities, it seems clear that NK cells and cytotoxic T8 cells share a common ancestry and fulfill the same xenophobic function of assaulting any cell, native or foreign, that presents false HLA credentials or viral determinants. Conceptual niceties are skirted by the descriptive term *large granular lymphocyte leukemia* (LGL-leukemia). As depicted in **Figure 44-1**, the "atypical lymphocytes" characteristic of this syndrome are nearly twice the size of normal lymphocytes, have bulky dark oblong nuclei, and are equipped with abundant blue-gray cytoplasm decorated with up to 20 red (azurophilic) granules. T8-CLL is an unusually languid clonal disorder. Disease begins with neutropenia and low white counts, which climb slowly as LGL numbers amplify, and a syndrome often emerges of neutropenia, recurrent infections, splenomegaly, and seropositive rheumatoid arthritis—a complex simulating Felty's syndrome. In LGL-leukemia with frank CD3+ T cell identification, white counts rarely exceed 20,000/μl and the course is so leisurely that harsh therapies are contraindicated. In LGL-leukemia with bold NK markers and absent or partial TcR rearrangements, the process may idle along for a few years as harmless lymphocytosis but eventually ignites into a malignant phase of marrow and nodal infiltration requiring chemotherapy.

Prolymphocytic leukemia (PLL) is a mortal affliction of the elderly marked by extreme lymphocytosis and pronounced splenomegaly but little or no adenopathy. This aggressive process is a leukemia of fully outfitted B cells *(immunoblasts)* and frequently arises as a *prolymphocytoid transformation* of B-CLL, as illustrated in **Figure 44-2** (×1,260). The 3 to 4 largest cells project the unmistakable image of immunoblasts: large round cells with dark blue cytoplasm, moderately condensed purple chromatin, and a single, centroidal, medallion-like nucleolus. This bold nucleolar navel can be obscured in cells shrivelled by shrinkage artifact, emphasizing the eternal imprecation to seek out well-spread areas. The 2 smaller cells in the upper left of this field, 1 having a tiny nucleolus, are remnants of the pre-existing CLL. A morphologically identical but less common T cell subset of PLL (T-PLL) can be identified by demonstrating strong focal reaction patterns for acid phosphatase, a badge of T cell proliferations. Prognosis in T-PLL is even more forlorn than in B-PLL.

Human T cell leukemia/lymphoma virus (HTLV-I) is a type C retrovirus etiologically associated with *adult T cell lymphoma* (ATL) endemic to southwest Japan, the Caribbean, and southeastern United States. Although contagious, this "slow virus" is only feebly productive, but in some individuals HTLV-I infection eventually immortalizes T cells and launches a violent lymphoproliferative syndrome characterized by lymphadenopathy, hepatosplenomegaly, cutaneous infiltration, lytic bone lesions with hypercalcemia, and morbid invasion of marrow. Malignant transformation occurs through "monoclonal" integration of provirus into the DNA of T4 cells, converting them into Sézary-like lymphocytes with deeply indented cerebriform nuclei. On blood smears the malignant lymphocytosis features pleomorphic cells with knobby nuclear conformations (**Figure 44-3**, ×1,260). The 3 largest leukemic lymphocytes shown display the irregular, clenched lobulations typical of T cell nuclei. The largest cell (abutting the band neutrophil) is clearly hyperdiploid and has the cytologic features of a T cell immunoblastic lymphoma. Most patients present with T cell lymphoma, but nearly all terminate with acute T cell leukemia, as was true in this patient. The mild but generalized red cell targeting in this blood smear is a harmless reflection of the patient's hemoglobin C trait.

Nuclear cleavage is not a monopoly of B-CLL. The primitive B cells that dwell at the center of lymph follicles (follicular centroblasts) acquire deep nuclear cleavage as they mature to follicular centrocytes. The malignant counterpart of centrocytes, *follicular lymphomas*, constitute about 30% of *non-Hodgkin's lymphomas*. Although follicular lymphomas are low-grade (slow-growing) lymphoid cancers, the disease is almost always disseminated at presentation. Lymphoma cells often retain the wanderlust of normal lymphocytes, and occasionally numerous large lymphoma cells with cleaved nuclei circulate in the blood (**Figure 44-4**, ×2,000). Presence of large lymphoma cells (cleaved or uncleaved) in blood has long been designated *lymphosarcoma cell leukemia*, but *lymphoma cell leukemia* is more apt. Discovery of exotic-looking lymphoma cells in blood is guaranteed to attract an enthusiastic crowd of morphology devotees.

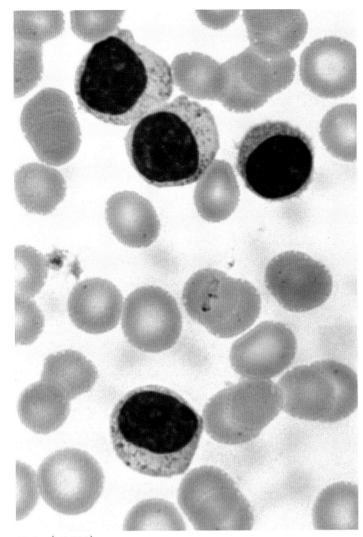

44-1 (×2,000)

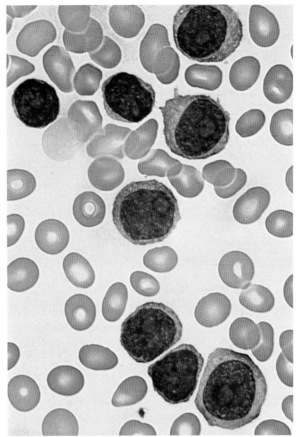

44-2 (×1,260)

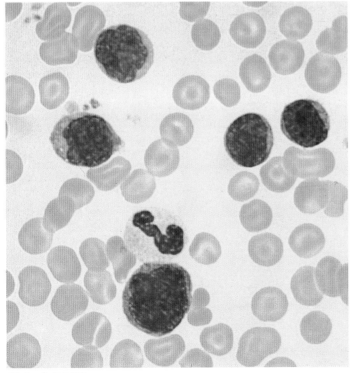

44-3 (×1,260)

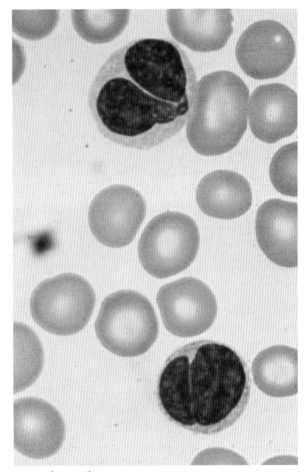

44-4 (×2,000)

Figure 45. Hairy Cell Leukemia

Hairy cell leukemia (HCL), formerly *leukemic reticuloendotheliosis,* originates as a lymphoma of mature splenic B cells (or, rarely, T cells), progresses to infiltrate the spleen and obliterate marrow, and eventually surfaces as a chronic leukemia. The inelegant name of this plodding proliferation affecting middle-aged men derives from the peculiar bristly appearance of hairy cell cytoplasm (**Figure 45-1,** ×2,000). Leukemic hairy cells project long shaggy or villous processes that determine many features of the disease and are key to the diagnosis. The cytoplasmic projections vary enormously from cell to cell and patient to patient. As illustrated by the antic trio in **Figure 45-1,** hairy cells may sport a frenetic wig, extend a bedraggled tuft or 2, or appear only faintly ruffled. All 3 cells shown are large for lymphocytes (15 to 18 μm across) and possess round or indented nuclei darkly filled with evenly condensed chromatin containing vague nucleoli.

In blood smears nuclear aberrations are upstaged by the intriguing, often comic cytoplasmic processes. In fixed tissue sections of infiltrated spleen, lymph nodes, or marrow, nuclear detail and heterogeneity are much more obvious. Spleen is extensively infiltrated early in HCL, and spleen sections stained with PAS-hematoxylin are particularly suitable for revealing nuclear configurations because red cells are unstained and the uncluttered tumor cell boundaries are thrown into relief. **Figure 45-4** (×1,260), which is stained in this manner, reveals a confectionery assortment of round, oblong, blocky, angular, reniform, coffee bean–shaped, clefted, and bisected nuclear variants. Basically these diverse contours can be classified into 3 kinds: ovoid, convoluted, and indented. The number of deeply indented or fissured nuclei and the fraction of cells with single bold nucleoli generally corresponds well with the geographic extent of marrow infiltration and hence the severity of pancytopenia and overt leukemia.

Disease expression in HCL can be attributed in part to the physical structure of hairy cells. Tumor infiltrates are kept spaced apart by the long cytoplasmic projections (although these prickly processes are nearly invisible in fixed sections). Consequently tumor cells appear much less tightly packed than is typical of lymphocytic proliferation, and tumor masses in spleen and nodes are proportionally bulkier. Examined at low power (**Figure 45-4**), solid tumor infiltrates appear pale and polka-dotted rather than dark and crammed. In marrow hairy cells become trapped and interlocked by their own spidery processes. Marrow contents often become gridlocked by the tightly knit tumor cells, and dry taps reward most efforts at marrow aspiration. As in spleen and nodes, hairy cells in marrow appear less crammed than in most leukemias and lymphomas because of wide nuclear spacing by the pale cytoplasmic processes. Frequently, marrow structural compression by infiltrates of HCL obliterates normal endothelial sinuses, which are replaced by small blood lakes or *pseudosinuses* containing red cells and surrounded by edema, as shown in an H&E-fixed section (**Figure 45-5,** ×1,260).

Most HCL patients are pancytopenic at presentation, and the percentage of hairy cells in blood is low. Even in advanced cases, white counts seldom exceed 25,000 cells/μl, a more usual figure being 10,000. Marrow replacement by tumor cells almost always leads to thrombocytopenia, and both neutropenia and severe monocyte depletion are constant features, undermining host resistance and predisposing to recurrent infections, the bête noir of HCL patients. Diagnosis can be inferred from the unique infiltrative pattern found in biopsy material, but proof depends on identifying individual tumor cells obtained from blood or (when hairy cells are infrequent) buffy coat preparations. Apart from their villous

or serrated cytoplasm, hairy cells can be distinguished from other leukemic lymphocytes by a unique combination of features: (1) tartrate-resistant acid phosphatase; (2) strong expression of IL-2 receptors (CD25, the "Tac" antigen); and (3) expression of monoclonal sIg, usually sIgG. Acid phosphatase activity, as indicated by red granular precipitates, is expressed weakly in normal lymphocytes but gives strong focal reaction products in most T cell leukemias and in HCL, even though most HCLs are B cell neoplasms. Unlike the isozymes 1 through 4 found in T cells, the isozyme 5 of hairy cells is uniquely insensitive to inhibition by tartrate, and demonstration of tartrate-resistant acid phosphatase (TRAP) activity in suspect lymphocytes is the most popular (but imperfect) diagnostic test for HCL. As depicted in **Figure 45-2** (×2,000), TRAP activity typically results in bright red focal deposits that hug the nucleus. This figure underscores the fact that some equally hirsute tumor cells are TRAP-negative; in patients with established HCL, only about half the hairy cells display this enzyme marker, and in 5% of patients none of the tumor cells are TRAP-positive. Variability in TRAP staining is borne out in **Figure 45-3** (×2,000), where 1 hairy cell contains heavy dye reaction products that are smeared brightly throughout the cytoplasm, but the other lacks any enzyme activity. Note, for comparison, the characteristically intense staining of platelets. TRAP-stained hairy cells can be counterstained with methyl green for nuclear emphasis, but these complementary dyes deaden each other and the extra manipulation may mat down the "hairs." TRAP activity has long been considered the trademark of HCL, but it is also expressed in exceptional cases of infectious mononucleosis, CLL, PLL, and Sézary syndrome. TRAP staining usually is not necessary for diagnosis of HCL.

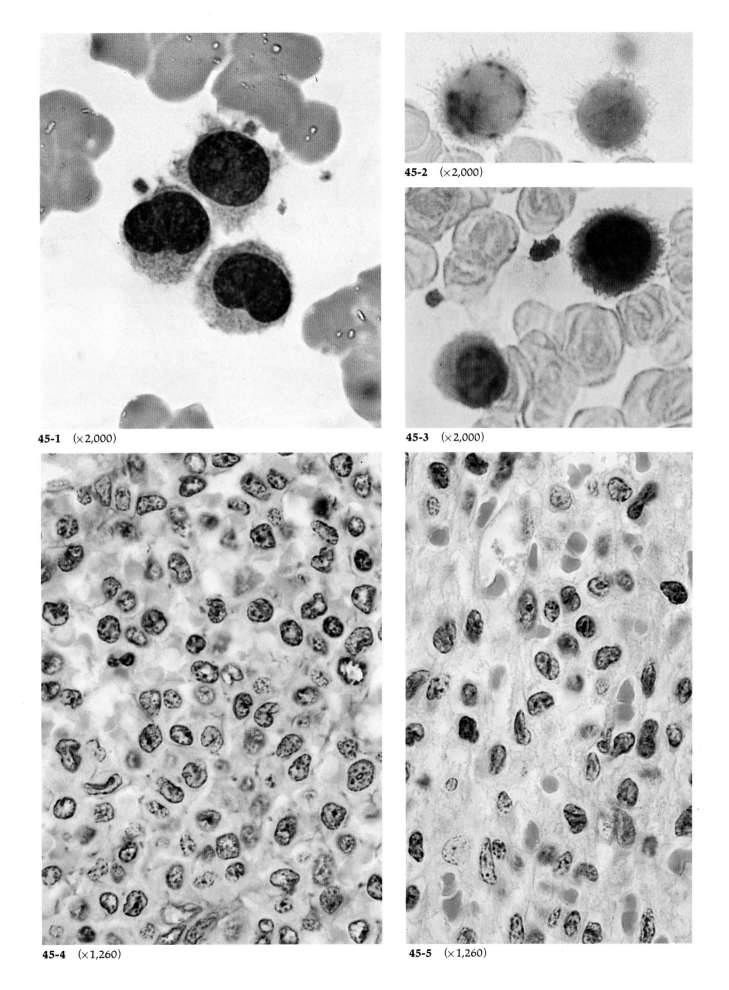

45-1 (×2,000)

45-2 (×2,000)

45-3 (×2,000)

45-4 (×1,260)

45-5 (×1,260)

Bibliography

Hematopoietic Malignancies

Appelbaum FR et al: Treatment of preleukemic syndromes with marrow transplantation. Blood 69 : 92, 1987

Bagby GC Jr: The concept of preleukemia: clinical and laboratory studies. CRC Crit Rev Oncol Hematol 4 : 203, 1986

Bishop JM: The molecular genetics of cancer. Science 235 : 305, 1987

Boice JD et al: Second cancers following radiation treatment for cervical cancer: an international collaboration among cancer registries. JNCI 74 : 955, 1985

Brodeur GM: Molecular correlates of cytogenetic abnormalities in human cancer cells: implications for oncogene activation. Prog Hematol 14 : 229, 1986

Doll R and Peto R: The Causes of Cancer. Oxford, Oxford University Press, 1981

Fox SB et al: Megakaryocytes in myelodysplasia: an immunohistochemical study on bone marrow trephines. Histopathology 17 : 69, 1990

Henderson ES and Lister TA, Eds: Leukemia, 5th ed. Philadelphia, WB Saunders Company, 1990

Kawaguchi M et al: Comparative study of immunocytochemical staining versus Giemsa stain for detecting dysmegakaryopoiesis in myelodysplastic syndromes (MDS). Eur J Haematol 44 : 89, 1990

Land CE and Tokunaga M: Induction period, in Radiation Carcinogenesis: Epidemiology and Biological Significance, Boice JD Jr and Fraumeni JF Jr, Eds. New York, Raven Press, 1984

Linet MS: The Leukemias: Epidemiologic Aspects. New York, Oxford University Press, 1985

List AF et al: The myelodysplastic syndromes: biology and implications for management. J Clin Oncol 8 : 1424, 1990

Moloney WC: Radiogenic leukemia revisited. Blood 70 : 905, 1987

Pedersen-Bjergaard J and Philip P: Cytogenetic characteristics of therapy-related acute nonlymphocytic leukaemia, preleukaemia and acute myeloproliferative syndrome: correlation with clinical data for 61 consecutive cases. Br J Haematol 66 : 199, 1987

Silverberg E and Lubera JA: Cancer statistics, 1988. CA 38 : 5, 1988

Third MIC Cooperative Study Group: Recommendations for a morphologic, immunologic, and cytogenetic (MIC) working classification of the primary and therapy-related myelodysplastic disorders. Cancer Genet Cytogenet 32 : 1, 1988

Varmus H: Retroviruses. Science 240 : 1427, 1988

Young JL Jr and Pollock ES: Chapt 8, in Cancer Epidemiology and Prevention, Schottenfeld D and Fraumeni JF Jr, Eds. Springfield, Charles C. Thomas, Publisher, 1982

Yunis JJ et al: Refined chromosome study helps define prognostic subgroups in most patients with primary myelodysplastic syndrome and acute myelogenous leukemia. Br J Haematol 68 : 189, 1988

Acute Myelogenous Leukemia

Appelbaum FR et al: Chemotherapy v. marrow transplantation for adults with acute nonlymphocytic leukemia: a five-year follow-up. Blood 72 : 179, 1988

Bennett JM et al: Criteria for the diagnosis of acute leukemia of megakaryocyte lineage (M7). A report of the French-American-British Cooperative Group. Ann Intern Med 103 : 460, 1985

Champlin RE and Gale RP: Role of bone marrow transplantation in the treatment of hematologic malignancies and solid tumors: critical review of syngeneic, autologous, and allogeneic transplants. Cancer Treat Rep 68 : 145, 1984

Fialkow PJ et al: Clonal development, stem-cell differentiation, and clinical remissions in acute nonlymphocytic leukemia. N Engl J Med 317 : 468, 1987

Foucar K: Bone marrow examination in the diagnosis of acute and chronic leukemias. Hematol Oncol Clin North Am 2 : 567, 1988

Griffin JD and Lowenberg B: Clonogenic cells in acute myeloblastic leukemia. Blood 68 : 1185, 1986

Hayhoe FGJ and Quaglino D: Haematological Cytochemistry, 2nd ed. Edinburgh, Churchill Livingstone, 1988

Jandl JH: Chapt 21, in Blood: Textbook of Hematology. Boston, Little, Brown and Company, 1987

McGlave PB et al: Allogeneic bone marrow transplanation for acute nonlymphocytic leukemia in first remission. Blood 72 : 1512, 1988

Pearson EC et al: Ultrastructure and cytogenetics in seven cases of acute promyelocytic leukaemia (APL). Br J Haematol 63 : 247, 1986

Chronic Myeloproliferative Disorders

Apperley JF et al: Bone marrow transplantation for chronic myeloid leukaemia in first chronic phase: importance of a graft-versus-leukaemia effect. Br J Haematol 69 : 239, 1988

Barnett MJ et al: An overview of bone marrow transplantation for chronic myeloid leukaemia. Can Med Assoc J 143 : 187, 1990

Bernstein R: Cytogenetics of chronic myelogenous leukemia. Semin Hematol 25 : 20, 1988

Champlin RE et al: Bone marrow transplantation in chronic myelogenous leukemia. Semin Hematol 25 : 74, 1988

Dokal I et al: Allogeneic bone marrow transplantation for primary myelofibrosis. Br J Haematol 71 : 158, 1989

Dreazen O et al: Molecular biology of chronic myelogenous leukemia. Semin Hematol 25 : 35, 1988

Ellis JT et al: Studies of the bone marrow in polycythemia vera and the evolution of myelofibrosis and second hematologic malignancies. Semin Hematol 23 : 144, 1986

Erslev AJ and Caro J: Pure erythrocytosis classified according to erythropoietin titers. Am J Med 76 : 57, 1984

Fenaux P et al: Clinical course of essential thrombocythemia in 147 cases. Cancer 66 : 549, 1990

Ferrant A: Chapter 6, in Myelofibrosis. Pathophysiology and Clinical Management, Lewis SM, Ed. New York, Marcel Dekker, Inc, 1985

Geary CG: Chapt 2, in Myelofibrosis. Pathophysiology and Clinical Management, Lewis SM, Ed. New York, Marcel Dekker, Inc, 1985

Goldman JM et al: Bone marrow transplantation for chronic myelogenous leukemia in chronic phase. Ann Intern Med 108 : 806, 1988

Hehlmann R et al: Essential thrombocythemia. Clinical characteristics and course of 61 cases. Cancer 61 : 2487, 1988

Iland HJ et al: Differentiation between essential thrombocythemia and polycythemia vera with marked thrombocytosis. Am J Hematol 25 : 191, 1987

Jandl JH: Chapt 22, in Blood: Textbook of Hematology. Boston, Little, Brown and Company, 1987

Juvonen E et al: Colony formation by megakaryocytic progenitors in essential thrombocythaemia. Br J Haematol 66 : 161, 1987

Kamada N and Uchino H: Chronologic sequence in appearance of clinical and laboratory findings characteristic of chronic myelocytic leukemia. Blood 51 : 843, 1978

Kaplan ME et al: Long-term management of polycythemia vera with hydroxyurea: a progress report. Semin Hematol 23 : 167, 1986

Kurzrock R et al: The molecular genetics of Philadelphia chromosome-positive leukemias. N Engl J Med 319 : 990, 1988

Leblond PF and Weed RI: The peripheral blood in polycythaemia vera and myelofibrosis. Clin Haematol 4 : 353, 1975

Schmidt U et al: Electron-microscopic characterization of mixed granulated (hybridoid) leucocytes of chronic myeloid leukaemia. Br J Haematol 68 : 175, 1988

Sokal JE et al: Staging and prognosis in chronic myelogenous leukemia. Semin Hematol 25 : 49, 1988

Spiers ASD: The clinical features of chronic granulocytic leukaemia. Clin Haematol 6 : 77, 1977

Stoll DB et al: Clinical presentation and natural history of patients with essential thrombocythemia and the Philadelphia chromosome. Am J Hematol 27 : 77, 1988

Talpaz M et al: Therapy of chronic myelogenous leukemia: chemotherapy and interferons. Semin Hematol 25 : 62, 1988

Wolf BC and Neiman RS: Myelofibrosis with myeloid metaplasia: pathophysiologic implications of the correlation between bone marrow changes and progression of splenomegaly. Blood 65 : 803, 1985

Acute Lymphatic Leukemia

Bloomfield CD et al: Chromosomal abnormalities and their clinical significance in acute lymphoblastic leukemia. Third International Workshop on Chromosomes in Leukemia. Cancer Res 43 : 868, 1983

Champlin R and Gale RP: Bone marrow transplantation for acute leukemia: recent advances and comparison with alternative therapies. Semin Hematol 24 : 55, 1987

Greaves MF and Chan LC: Is spontaneous mutation the major 'cause' of childhood acute lymphoblastic leukaemia? Br J Haematol 64 : 1, 1986

Greaves MF et al: Differentiation-linked gene rearrangement and expression in acute lymphoblastic leukaemia. Clin Haematol 15 : 621, 1986

Hara J et al: Relationship between rearrangement and transcription of the T-cell receptor α,β, and γ genes in B-precursor acute lymphoblastic leukemia. Blood 73 : 500, 1989

Kass L and Elias JM: Cytochemistry and immunocytochemistry in bone marrow examination: contemporary techniques for the diagnosis of acute leukemia and myelodysplastic syndromes. A combined approach. Hematol Oncol Clin North Am 2 : 537, 1988

Kurtzberg J et al: CD7+, CD4-,CD8- acute leukemia: a syndrome of malignant pluripotent lymphohematopoietic cells. Blood 73 : 381, 1989

LeBien TW and McCormack RT: The common acute lymphoblastic leukemia antigen (CD10)—emancipation from a functional enigma. Blood 73 : 625, 1989

Proctor SJ et al: A comparative study of combination chemotherapy versus marrow transplant in first remission in adult acute lymphoblastic leukaemia. Br J Haematol 69 : 35, 1988

Chronic Lymphatic Leukemia and Related Disorders

Bertoli LF et al: Analysis with antiidiotype antibody of a patient with chronic lymphocytic leukemia and a large cell lymphoma (Richter's syndrome). Blood 70 : 45, 1987

Binet JL et al: A new prognostic classification of chronic lymphocytic leukemia derived from a multivariate survival analysis. Cancer 48 : 198, 1981

Bunn PA Jr: Clinical features in T-cell lymphoproliferative syndrome associated with human T-cell leukemia/lymphoma virus, Broder S, moderator. Ann Intern Med 100 : 543, 1984

Costello C et al: Prolymphocytic leukaemia: an untrastructural study of 22 cases. Br J Haematol 44 : 389, 1980

Deegan MJ et al: High incidence of monoclonal proteins in the serum and urine of chronic lymphocytic leukaemia. Blood 64 : 1207, 1984

Feliu E et al: Cytoplasmic inclusions in lymphocytes of chronic lymphocytic leukaemia. Scand J Haematol 31 : 510, 1983

French Cooperative Group on Chronic Lymphocytic Leukemia: Prognostic and therapeutic advances in CLL management: the experience of the French Cooperative Group. Semin Hematol 24 : 275, 1987

Golomb HM et al: "Hairy" cell leukaemia (leukaemic reticuloendotheliosis): a scanning electron microscopic study of eight cases. Br J Haematol 29 : 455, 1975

Golomb HM and Ratain MJ: Recent advances in the treatment of hairy-cell leukaemia. N Engl J Med 316 : 870, 1987

Greaves MF et al: Chapt 9, in Atlas of Blood Cells: Function and Pathology, vol. 1, Zucker-Franklin D et al, Eds. Milan, Edi. Ermes s.r.l., 1988

Grem JL et al: Pentostatin in hairy cell leukemia: treatment by the special exception mechanism. JNCI 81 : 448, 1989

Henderson ES and Lister TA, Eds: Leukemia, 5th ed. Philadelphia, WB Saunders Company, 1990

Jaffe ES et al: The pathologic spectrum of adult T-cell leukemia/lymphoma in the United States. Am J Surg Pathol 8 : 263, 1984

Jandl JH: Chapt 25, in Blood: Textbook of Hematology. Boston, Little, Brown and Company, 1987

Kay NE and Perri RT: Evidence that large granular lymphocytes from B-CLL patients with hypogammaglobulinemia down-regulate B-cell immunoglobulin synthesis. Blood 73 : 1016, 1989

Kruskall MS and Harris NL: Chronic lymphocytic leukemia with the recent development of hepatosplenomegaly and ascites. Case 31-1983. N Engl J Med 309 : 297, 1983.

Matutes E et al: The morphological spectrum of T-prolymphocytic leukaemia. Br J Haematol 64 : 111, 1986

Melo JV et al: The relationship between chronic lymphocytic leukaemia and prolymphocytic leukaemia. IV. Analysis of survival and prognostic features. Br J Haematol 65 : 23, 1987

Montserrat E et al: Lymphocyte doubling time in chronic lymphocytic leukaemia: analysis of its prognostic signficance. Br J Haematol 62 : 567, 1986

Salahuddin SZ et al: Isolation of a new virus, HBLV, in patients with lymphoproliferative disorders. Science 234 : 596, 1986

Sheridan W et al: Leukemia of non-T lineage natural killer cells. Blood 72 : 1701, 1988

Sweet DL Jr et al: Chronic lymphocytic leukaemia and its relationship to other lymphoproliferative disorders. Clin Haematol 6 : 141, 1977

Turner A and Kjeldsberg CR: Hairy cell leukemia: a review. Medicine 57 : 477, 1978

Wachsman W et al: HTLV and human leukemia: perspectives 1986. Semin Hematol 24 : 245, 1986

V. Plasma Cell Malignancies

Multiple Myeloma and Macroglobulinemia

Figure 46. Multiple Myeloma

Multiple myeloma (plasma cell myeloma, plasmacytoma), a differentiated B cell neoplasm, is a solid tumor having more in common with lymphoma than leukemia. Tumor masses usually appear first within marrow and continue to show a strong and destructive tropism for marrow during their dissemination, cropping up throughout the skeleton to form multiple osteolytic lesions. Invading myeloma cells secrete monoclonal immunoglobulins *(M components)* and a brew of self-serving cytokines that collectively suppress synthesis of normal immunoglobulins, inhibit hematopoiesis, and activate osteoclasts to corrode bone and create tumor spaces. The net result is a devastating syndrome of successive calamities that include pathologic fractures, hypercalcemia, renal impairment, recurrent infections, and marrow failure. Patients commonly present with a pathologic fracture or abrupt collapse of a vertebra associated with moderately severe, nondescript normocytic anemia. The first clues to diagnosis may be the prosaic discovery of prominent rouleaux and heavy background discoloration in Wright-Giemsa stained blood smears (**Figure 46-1,** ×200). Red cells stack up into rouleaux, some of which exhibit bifurcative branchings, because of the high concentrations of monoclonal immunoglobulin. Coarse rouleaux, whether caused by a clonal M component, a polyclonal immunoglobulin rise, or elevated fibrinogen, interfere with preparation of well-spread smears, a problem easily solved by diluting anticoagulated blood with saline. The diffuse pinkish gray background staining in **Figure 46-1** was caused by the heavy film of dried immunoglobulin *paraprotein*. Presence of hyperglobulinemic staining is affirmed by the clear window at the upper left, where stained protein was rubbed off during preparation.

Myeloma cells vary considerably from patient to patient, and there is a crude correspondence between the degree of atypia in plasma cells and their biologic belligerence. In **Figure 46-2** (×800), myeloma cells are of mixed appearance. Most tumor cells are small normal-looking plasma cells with blue-gray mottled cytoplasm, dark and muddied at the margins, and with well-condensed eccentric nuclei. Many of these otherwise friendly-appearing cells possess 1 or 2 small nucleoli as badges of aggression. More dangerous still are the larger cells, several of them binucleate, with immature nuclei, finely divided chromatin, and prominent, pale, single nucleoli. These are *plasmablasts,* and their presence in large numbers conveys a dismal prognosis. Nearly all cells in **Figure 46-3** (×1,260) are exemplary, robust-looking mature plasma cells, with nuclei eccentric and cytoplasm in heraldic color. This population is characteristic of plasmacytic (as opposed to plasmablastic) myeloma; in this "more favorable" form of myeloma, survival is superior (up to several years), but the extended years are darkened by a dispiriting crescendo of pain and disability. Accurate prognostic staging is complicated by the admixture, in most patients, of varying proportions of mature and plasmablastic forms and by the morphologic variability created when crowded areas of slides are compared with areas more open to scrutiny. When plasma cells occur in swarms or sheets, as in **Figures 46-2** and **46-3,** diagnosis of myeloma is not in doubt. If the proportion of plasma cells is in the 10 to 20% range, the finding of nonrandom clusters of plasma cells is an important indicator that the cells are malignant. Even when geographic occupation of marrow by myeloma is extensive, leukoerythroblastic reactions are curiously subdued, and relatively few myeloma cells enter the bloodstream. An exception to this is a rampaging disorder known as *plasma cell leukemia* in which myeloma cell levels in blood average about 30,000/μl and monoclonal IgE is overrepresented.

The most diagnostic and stage-related feature of myeloma is release into serum or urine of a single homogeneous immunoglobulin or immunoglobulin fragment. Myeloma cells display Ig gene rearrangements that take place after Ig class switching, and hence all classes of monoclonal Ig are represented and occur in approximate correspondence to their normal fractional synthetic rates. More than half of patients have IgG myeloma, about 25% have IgA myeloma, and IgD, IgE, and IgM myelomas are uncommon. Light chain and heavy chain secretion is unbalanced in most patients, and in more than 10% of cases the only gene product is free light chains *(Bence Jones protein)*. Abnormalities of Ig production and secretion lead to intracytoplasmic deposits of immunoglobulin that plug and dilate the Golgi cisternae. Dense spherical accumulations of immunoglobulin may agglomerate within individual plasma cells, causing them to resemble bunches of grapes. These *grape cells* or *morular forms* are most widely known as *Mott cells* (**Figure 46-4,** ×2,000). Mott cells are a characteristic but not unique feature of myeloma. They occur also in polyclonal hyperglobulinemic disorders, indicating that Mott cells represent obstipation from Ig overload rather than a primary malignant change.

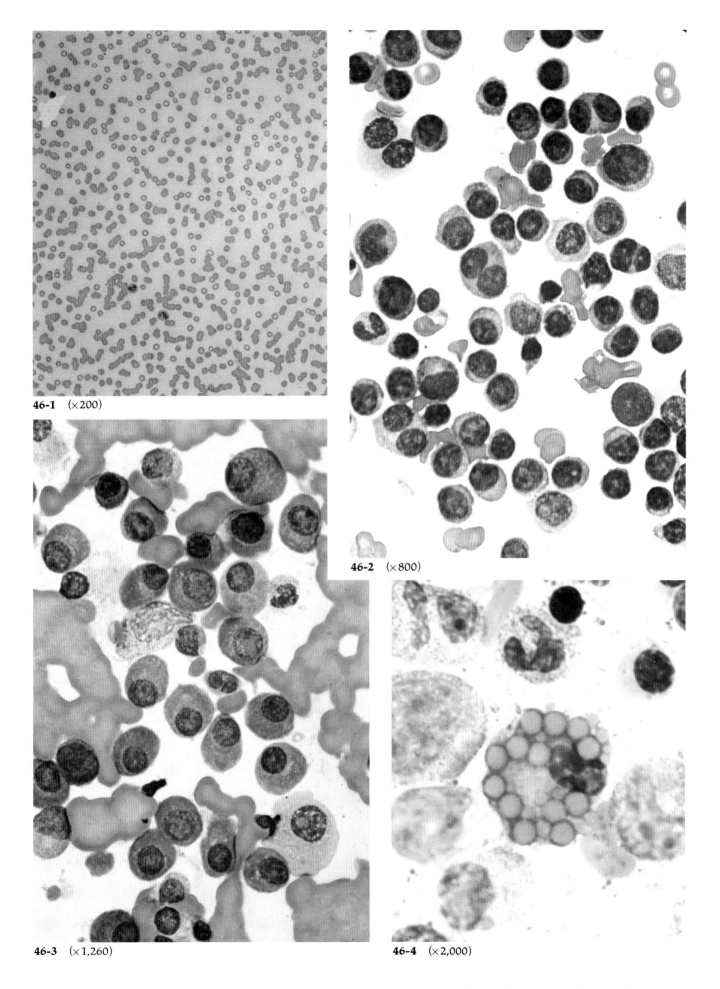

46-1　(×200)

46-2　(×800)

46-3　(×1,260)

46-4　(×2,000)

Figure 47. Multiple Myeloma: Cytologic Art and Oddities. Waldenström's Macroglobulinemia.

Derangements of immunoglobulin synthesis and secretion in malignant plasma cells are responsible for a museumlike assortment of cytologic aberrations. Among the most dazzling are giant multinucleated plasma cells with fiery fringes known as *flaming cells* (**Figure 47-1,** ×1,260). The heavy magenta or carmine coloring of the margins of these dysplastic but picturesque forms is caused by plugging of peripheral secretory channels by precipitated immunoglobulin or immunoglobulin fragments. Secretory obstruction devitalizes and thickens cell margins, eventually causing the dying cell to shed hardened fragments of cytoplasm. Some flaming cells take on a strange and startling beauty, like miniature oriental rugs. Plasma cells with flamed borders are most common in IgA myeloma, but identical cells can be found in other myelomas and similar forms occasionally appear during reactive plasmacytosis. Flaming cells are not designed to be storage cells, for they lack the digestive enzymes to assimilate their surfeit of immunoglobulin. True storage macrophages, laden with sphingolipids released by the dying multitudes of plasma cells, are common in myeloma infiltrates; these sphingolipid-fattened macrophages may acquire the bulky tigroid look of Gaucher cells, as indicated in **Figure 38-4**.

Much more common in myeloma than flaming cells or Gaucherlike cells are plasma cells filled with dense spherical immunoglobulin inclusions, such as those seen in Mott cells (see **Figure 46-4**). Unbalanced immunoglobulin synthesis is responsible for an assortment of pink, blue, or colorless inclusions. These include hyaline cytoplasmic spherules known as *Russell bodies* and their intranuclear counterparts (intranuclear dense bodies). When occurring in small numbers or singly (**Figure 47-3,** ×2,000), Russell bodies appear cherry red and may be several μm across. These showy inclusions, which are PAS-positive, are found also in chronic inflammatory disorders and thus are not emblems of malignant change. Among other inclusions created by faulty biosynthesis in malignant or reactive plasma cells are spindle-shaped azurophilic crystals of immunoglobulin (**Figure 47-4,** ×1,260). Some of these rigid, needle-sharp structures are dislodged during the washing procedure, leaving behind their vacated silhouettes.

It is unusual for plasma cells to engage in activities other than manufacture and secretion of immunoglobulin. In exceptional cases myeloma cells may phagocytize red cells and neutrophils, as shown in **Figure 47-2** (×1,260), as well as platelets. Phagocytic myeloma cells appear properly differentiated, and the explanation for this odd appetite is unknown.

Waldenström's macroglobulinemia (WM) is an indolent secretory B cell malignancy manifested by accumulation of monoclonal IgM in plasma, lymphadenopathy, hepatosplenomegaly, and invasion of marrow and nodes by plasmacytoid lymphocytes (**Figure 47-5,** ×1,260). Infiltrates contain a disorderly mixture of lymphocytes, plasma cells, and large numbers of lymphoid cells intermediate in appearance—hybrid cells known in hematologic argot as *plymphs*. The polymorphic, motley (not Mottly) appearance of tumor cell infiltrates explains heavy reliance on the fudge ending "-oid" so often used in descriptions of WM cytology. The range of heterogeneity and heavy representation by conventional looking plasma cells and lymphocytes is well shown in **Figure 47-5**, as is the surplus stroma and an eye-catching mast cell. Despite their morphologic heterogeneity, the lymphs, plymphs, and plasma cells comprising WM infiltrates are all members of the same clone, and their clonal IgM class places the point of stem cell mutation at a level just prior to the heavy chain class switch. *Tissue mast cells* are characteristic and numerous in WM marrow but

are present as reactive onlookers, not being members of the B cell clone. Mast cells are of macrophage provenance and can be distinguished from their circulating myeloid analogues, basophils, by their larger size, heavier load of metachromatic granules, and pale round nucleus. Clinical features of WM stem from high levels of monoclonal IgM, molecules of which are confined by their girth to the plasma compartment, where they exert an unbalanced transendothelial osmotic force leading to hypervolemia as well as hyperviscosity. Increased blood volume and viscosity combine to exhaust the myocardium, disturb mentation, gum up peripheral nerves, and plug glomeruli. Dilutional anemia is invariable, usually complicated by blood loss from engorged mucosal surfaces. Consequently, red cells are commonly hypochromic and form striking rouleaux, with a proportionate increase in sedimentation rates. Leukocytosis is uncommon, but the monoclonal nature of lymphoplasmacytoid cells in blood and marrow can be certified by *kappa/lambda analysis* of cellular surface membrane immunoglobulin.

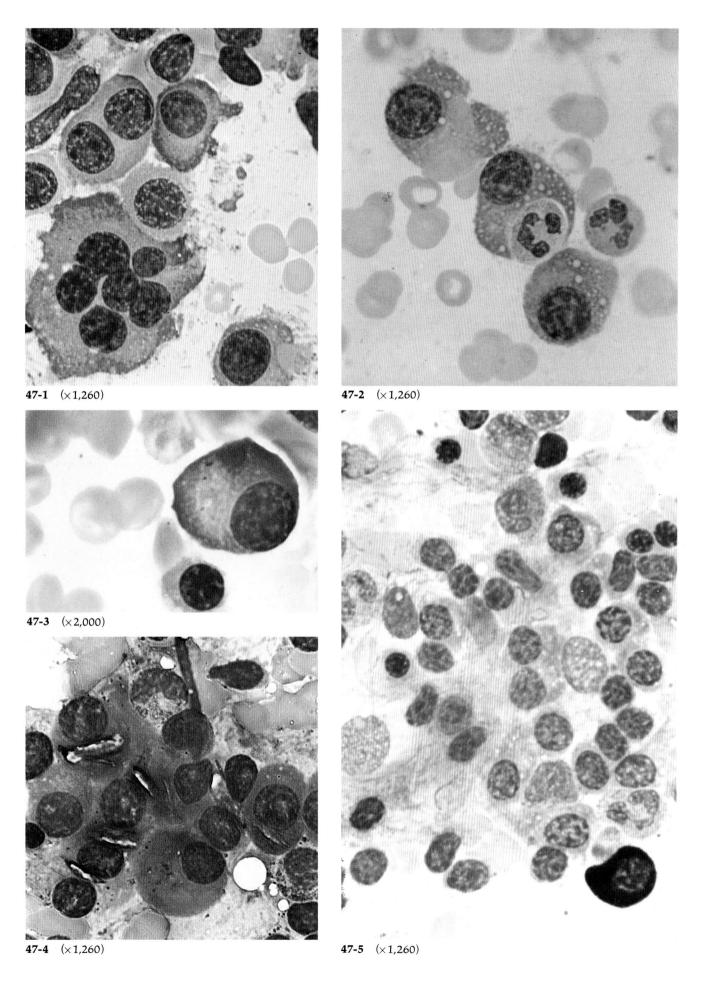

47-1 (×1,260)

47-2 (×1,260)

47-3 (×2,000)

47-4 (×1,260)

47-5 (×1,260)

Bibliography

Multiple Myeloma and Macroglobulinemia

Azar HA: Chapt 1, in Multiple Myeloma and Related Disorders, vol. I, Azar HA and Potter M, Eds. New York, Harper & Row, Publishers, Inc, 1973

Barlogie B et al: Plasma cell myeloma—new biological insights and advances in therapy. Blood 73 : 865, 1989

Bartl R et al: Bone marrow histology in Waldenstrom's macroglobulinaemia. Clinical relevance of subtype recognition. Scand J Haematol 31 : 359, 1983

Bartl R et al: Histologic classification and staging of multiple myeloma: a retrospective and prospective study of 674 cases. Am J Clin Pathol 87 : 342, 1987

Bartl R et al: Bone marrow histology and serum beta 2 microglobulin in multiple myeloma—a new prognostic strategy. Eur J Haematol (Suppl 51)43 : 88, 1989

Coward RA: Chapt 16, in Multiple Myeloma and Other Paraproteinemias, Delamore IN, Ed. Edinburgh, Churchill Livingstone, 1986

Gahrton G et al: Allogeneic bone marrow transplantation in 24 patients with multiple myeloma reported to the EBMT registry. Hematol Oncol 6: 181, 1988

Gould J et al: Plasma cell karyotype in multiple myeloma. Blood 71 : 453, 1988

Hayhoe FGJ et al: Chapt 6, in Multiple Myeloma and Other Paraproteinemias, Delamore IN, Ed. Edinburgh, Churchill Livingstone, 1986

Jandl JH: Chapt 26, in Blood: Textbook of Hematology. Boston, Little, Brown and Company, 1987

Johns EA et al: Isoelectric points of urinary light chains in myelomatosis: analysis in relation to nephrotoxicity. J Clin Pathol 39 : 833, 1986

Kyle RA and Greipp PR: The laboratory investigation of monoclonal gammopathies. Mayo Clin Proc 53 : 719, 1978

Kyle RA: 'Benign' monoclonal gammopathy: a misnomer? JAMA 251 : 1849, 1984

Merlini G et al: Monoclonal immunoglobulins with antibody activity in myeloma, macroglobulinemia and related plasma cell dyscrasias. Semin Oncol 13 : 350, 1986

Osserman EF et al: Multiple myeloma and related plasma cell dyscrasias. JAMA 258 : 2930, 1987

Paladini G: Chapter 13, in Multiple Myeloma and Other Paraproteinemias, Delamore IN, Ed. Edinburgh, Churchill Livingstone, 1986

Riches PG: Chapt 5, in Multiple Myeloma and Other Paraproteinemias, Delamore IN, Ed. Edinburgh, Churchill Livingstone, 1986

Seligmann M et al: Heavy chain diseases: current findings and concepts. Immunol Rev 48 : 145, 1979

Weinstein T et al: Electron microscopy study of Mott and Russell bodies in myeloma cells. J Submicrosc Cytol 19 : 155, 1987

Zukerberg LR et al: Plasma cell myeloma with cleaved, multilobated, and monocytoid nuclei. Am J Clin Pathol 93 : 657, 1990

VI. Lymphomas

Figures 48 through 51. Introduction to Lymphomas

Lymphomas are solid malignant tumors of the lymphoreticular system. Distinction between leukemias and lymphomas rests on geographic grounds, leukemias arising from marrow and freely trespassing the marrow : blood barrier, lymphomas originating in primary or secondary lymphoid tissues and only occasionally venturing into the bloodstream. Lymphomas, collectively the most prevalent hematopoietic neoplasms, are grouped into 2 very different families. *Hodgkin's disease* comprises a strangely polymorphic collection of nodal tumors united under the emblem of a numinous giant cell known as the *Reed-Sternberg* (RS) *cell*. *Non-Hodgkin's lymphomas* (NHLs) constitute an intimidating and extended family of lymphoid tumors, encompassing diverse B cell malignancies of lymph node follicles and several less common T cell proliferations, plus a smattering of macrophage malignancies.

Hodgkin's disease (HD) originates in lymph nodes and disseminates by direct extension. The neoplastic clonal founder cell and logo of HD, the exotic and the enigmatic RS cell, is vastly outnumbered in tumor cell populations by a disorderly polyclonal rabble of lymphocytes, eosinophils, and plasma cells. The impression conveyed is of guerrilla warfare, not of the regimented invasions characteristic of cancer. Indeed, this rebellious histology and the elusive phenotypy of RS cells have long encouraged the view that HD is an infective reaction, but in all essentials HD behaves as a true neoplasm, growing out of control, infiltrating vital organs, and submitting only to tumoricidal agents. The annual new case incidence of HD in the United States is 7,400, with about 1,500 fatalities. This implies an overall mortality of 20%, a tribute to combined modality therapy. Unlike other malignancies, including NHLs, HD incidence is bimodal, with an early peak at age 20 to 30 and a second summit after age 60.

The diverse histopathology of HD is subdivided into 4 morphologically distinctive entities. HD tumors may display a favorable *lymphocyte predominance* pattern at one extreme and an unfavorable (and happily less common) *lymphocyte depletion* histology at the other. Almost half of cases show a picturesque process in which tumor cells are encased by *nodular sclerosis*, usually intimating localized disease. Another 25% are characterized by *mixed cellularity*, which conveys an intermediate prognosis. HD presents as painless asymmetrical enlargement of nodes above the diaphragm, followed by a pattern of contiguous axial spread. Systemic symptoms are portentous prognostic indicators, denoted in staging classifications by the suffixed letter B: the *B triad* consists of fever, night sweats, and loss of 10% or more of weight in the prior 6 months. Diagnosis of HD (and of NHL) is made by histologic examination of excised nodes. When there is a choice, the largest lower cervical or axillary lymph node is removed intact and sent immediately to the pathology laboratory. Before formalin fixation, a portion of suspect tissue is frozen for subsequent cell marker studies, flow cytometry, chromosome studies, and viral cultures.

Non-Hodgkin's lymphomas are far more common than HD, with more than 35,000 new cases diagnosed annually in the United States and the number rising steeply with the advent of the AIDS era and as the penalty for immunosuppressive pharmaceuticals. Several consecutive steps are operative in fomenting NHLs in patients immunosuppressed by HIV infection or by chemotherapy used for transplant recipients: sabotage of T cells; escape of latent Epstein-Barr virus (EBV) infection; and, eventually, appearance of clonal chromosomal abnormalities. Most NHLs are B cell neoplasms occurring as clonal transformations reflecting specific stages of B cell differentiation in lymphatic follicles. *Follicular lymphomas*, with growth patterns that possess some resemblance to normal nodal architecture, are more indolent than are *diffuse lymphomas*, which lack structure and insinuate aggression. Approximately 85% of lymphomas with follicular (nodal) morphology are associated with a clonal t(14;18) chromosomal translocation, affirming the single cell origin of the tumor. The B cell clonal origin of most lymphomas can also be certified by demonstration of *immunoglobulin gene rearrangements*, amplified when necessary by *polymerase chain reaction* (PCR) technology. In the western hemisphere about 15% of NHLs are of T cell origin, as determined by T cell markers and clonal gene rearrangements of the TcR. T cell lymphomas of thymic provenance share many features with T cell ALL, including diffuse pattern of spread, knobby nuclei, TdT positivity, mediastinal presentation, and poor prognosis.

Classification of NHLs lacking the RS logo is characterized by colossal confusion. In a commendable quest for harmony, a group of lymphoma grandees has devised a *"Working Formulation"* (WF) that is slowly falling into favor. WF terminology and equivalent terms employed in the deplored but durable Rappaport classification are used in the ensuing descriptions. In reading lymphoma literature, readers should bear in mind that in the Rappaport system, "nodular" means "follicular" and "histiocyte" stands for many things, including transformed lymphocytes and macrophages. Basically, ongoing classifications segregate NHLs into low-, intermediate-, and high-grade categories that predict survival of 5 to 7 years, 2 to 5 years, and less than 2 years, respectively. The grim irony of lymphoma grading is that nearly 50% of patients with high-grade NHLs respond lastingly to intensive chemotherapy, whereas low-grade lymphomas progress slowly but resist eradication and eventually (within about 10 years) transform to high-grade histology.

Figure 48. Hodgkin's Disease

Reed-Sternberg (RS) cells are the insignia of Hodgkin's disease and are central to the diagnosis. On Wright-Giemsa stained smears of marrow aspirates (**Figures 48-1,** ×800 and **48-2,** ×1,260), classic RS cells are very large and possess voluminous pale blue-gray cytoplasm surrounding 2 or more oval nuclei, each of which contains an immense nucleolus. No other morphologic finding in hematology has the mystique accorded the RS cell. It is the totem and touchstone of Hodgkin's disease (HD), searched for amid lymphoidal proliferations by thousands of hematopathologists each and every day. Marrow is not the best place for seeking this talismanic cell, for only in advanced disease do RS cells disseminate so far from their nodal origins. HD ordinarily arises in lymph nodes, and the largest suspect node is the place to look. HD is a disease of exceptions, and one of these is that RS cells are most obvious on H&E–stained sections. In sections the RS cell in its several variant forms is notable for the startling *inclusion body* appearance of its nucleoli. Even in the smaller bilobate variant nuclei found in nodular sclerosis, the owlish binocular glare of the purple nucleoli has a demonic cast (**Figure 48-4,** ×800). Identification of RS cells is a commitment to use specified and risky therapeutic modalities, so it is imperative to sort out look-alike cells that can be encountered in reactive nodes containing activated T cells (for example, in infectious mononucleosis) as well as in large cell lymphoma and certain T cell lymphomas.

Diagnosis of HD depends on detecting RS cells in a compatible context. This means the giant cells must be found in the mixed company of malignant-looking macrophages or "histiocytes" *(H cells)* and a consortium of normal or mildly irregular lymphocytes, plasma cells, and eosinophils—all of which are visible in **Figures 48-1** and **48-4.** In H&E–stained sections, at least 4 variants of RS cells have been certified and these correlate roughly with histopathologic subsets of HD. In *lymphocyte predominant HD,* RS cells are sparse and occur amid multitudes of lymphocytes and numerous histiocytes *(L&H forms)*: these RS cells are hyperlobated *popcorn cells* possessing wrinkled or twisted nuclei and small nucleoli. Popcorn cells can be located more readily within the busy contours of the nucleus by use of methyl green pyronin stain, for the nucleoli are intensely pyroninophilic. In *nodular sclerosing HD* (**Figure 48-3,** ×200) RS *lacunar cells* are imprisoned within sclerotic chambers of connective tissue. Because of the discordant shrinkage artifacts that characterize sclerotic specimens after fixation, the bilobate or multinuclear RS cells stand out naked against the retracted pale cytoplasm, like bugs in amber (**Figure 48-4**). Note in **Figures 48-3** and **48-4** that there are few if any transitional or intermediate forms such as characterize infiltrates of NHLs; the giant RS cells are totally different in size and appearance from the sea of lymphocytes, plasma cells, and granulocytes that engulf them. Whether or not lacunar cells resemble classic RS cells, RS-like cells in this cocoonlike setting confer the imprimatur of HD. In the polymorphous infiltrates of *mixed cellularity HD,* classic binucleate or multinucleated RS cells are numerous and possess the most startling of all inclusionlike nucleoli. *Lymphocyte depletion HD,* the least common but most deadly form of HD, is marked by swarms of atypical RS and H cells, with only a few embattled lymphocytes remaining on the scene. The finding of macrophages with bold nucleoli in a Hodgkin's-like setting, or the discovery of giant pyknotic "zombie cells" with obscured cytology, should always prompt a determined search for diagnostic RS cells.

Molecular probe technology has not resolved the issue as to the lineage derivation of RS cells, partly because these intriguing giants are usually surrounded by an entourage of polyclonal helper T cells, admixed with variable collections of reactive onlookers, including B cells, plasma cells, and granulocytes. RS cells are comparatively populous in the prevalent nodular sclerosing and mixed cellular subsets of HD, and molecular genetic studies in enriched cellular populations derived from these tumors have revealed rearrangements of T cell receptor genes, of immunoglobulin genes, of both, and of neither. Both RS and H cells display the Ki-1, Leu-M1, and IL-2 receptor (Tac) antigens, but this phenotypic profile applies to activated cells of several lineages. Considering this and the macrophagelike look and behavior of RS cells, some lymphoma luminaries have championed the politic proposal that HD is a hybrid or chimeric tumor of mixed T cell and monocyte derivation. As was long inferred from histologic appearances, HD may be a family of distinctive lymphoid proliferations spawned in obedience to cytokines such as IL-1 released by the imperious RS founder cells. Happily, ignorance of pathogenesis has not deferred discovery that (in most cases) HD can be cured by combined modality therapy.

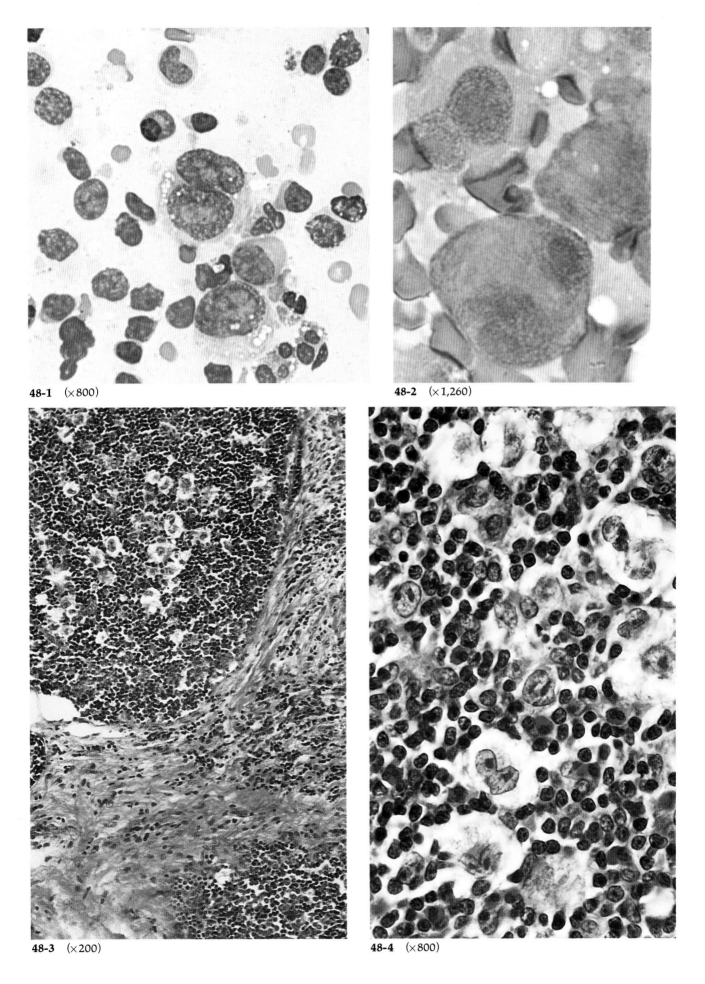

48-1 (×800)

48-2 (×1,260)

48-3 (×200)

48-4 (×800)

Figure 49. Non-Hodgkin's Lymphomas. Follicular Small Cleaved Cell Lymphoma. Diffuse Large Cell Lymphoma. (H&E–stained sections).

Non-Hodgkin's lymphomas are a complex group of distinctive clonal tumors that originate in lymphoid tissues. Most are malignant versions of cellular components of normal lymph nodes: hence, NHLs are mainly B cell tumors (80%), some (15%) bear T cell credentials, and a few stem from macrophages. Diagnosis is generally based on biopsy of enlarged peripheral nodes, but, unlike Hodgkin's disease, NHLs often appear first in small extranodal sites off the lymphoid mainstream. Patterns of growth and cell size are the vital determinants of tumor aggressiveness. Tumors that grow in *follicular (nodular) patterns* (**Figure 49-1,** ×200) have a distinctly better prognosis than *diffuse lymphomas* having unstructured growth (**Figure 49-2,** ×200). This difference fulfills the intuitive expectation that growth patterns possessing some resemblance to normal follicular architecture are more differentiated and less belligerent than diffuse, swarming, anarchic infiltrations. It bears repeating that in the lymphoma world the terms *nodular* and *follicular* are used interchangeably, even though *nodular* merely signifies small lumps whereas *follicular* connotes origins from or resemblance to the B cell follicles of lymph nodes. Indeed, all follicular lymphomas possess a B cell phenotype and show clonal immunoglobulin gene rearrangements, and the vast majority share a common, clonal, chromosomal motif—a 14;18 translocation. Diffuse lymphomas, in contrast, are heterogeneous, higher-grade malignancies derived from B cells, T cells, or macrophages, and display an assortment of phenotypic and genotypic markers.

Diffuse lymphomas are easily recognized as malignant by their unstructured growth. The histology of follicular lymphomas such as the *follicular small cleaved cell lymphoma* (nodular poorly differentiated lymphoma [NPDL]) depicted in **Figure 49-1** must be distinguished from that of reactive follicular hyperplasia. Benign reactive follicles contain a centroidal colony of basophilic B cell blasts *(centroblasts),* constituting a "dark zone," in which big, pale *tingible body macrophages* are interspersed, conferring "starry sky" imagery. Centroblasts are large, rapidly proliferating cells with plump nuclei containing 2 or more membrane-adherent nucleoli. As centroblasts migrate outward, they transform into placid cells with angular or cleaved nuclei and abundant pale cytoplasm; these *centrocytes* accumulate apart from the parental mass of centroblasts and create a "light zone." The entire germinal center structure, encompassing both the dark- and light-zone populations, plus the phagocytic tingible macrophages, is surrounded by a thick collar of close-packed B cells (and some T cells) known as the *mantle zone.* The foregoing literary excursion is meant to emphasize the organized design-work involved in reactive follicles. The nodular structures in **Figure 49-1** superficially resemble large lymphoid follicles and even possess mantle zones, but the enveloped tumor population is a random and disorganized assemblage of large cells (centroblasts) and smaller cleaved cells (centrocytes). There is no germinal center, no focus of mitotic activity, no tingible body macrophages, and no separation into dark zones and light zones. This is the histology of a follicular lymphoma. The motley composition of the tumor cell population shown in **Figure 49-1** is revealed at higher magnification in **Figure 49-3** (×1,260). The predominant cells possess dark angular nuclei, most of which are bent, creased, or folded. Amid these "cleaved cells" (centrocytes) are small numbers of large uncleaved cells (centroblasts) with potato-like nuclei and 2 or 3 nucleoli. In addition there are several bulky blast cells (transformed B cells) each having a single bold purple or pink nucleolus. The largeness of uncleaved cells connotes active cell cycling, whereas the collapsed angu-

lar look of centrocytes signifies a resting (G_0) state. Both populations, cleaved and uncleaved, stain for a single surface immunoglobulin isotype, indicating a common clonal origin. Absence of macrophages containing tingible bodies (pieces of phagocytized DNA) attests to the witless vigor of the tumor cells. Tingible body macrophages are a fixture of well-regulated follicles because of a necrophilic aspect of B cell reactions to antigens, known as *programmed cell death.* This physiologic reaction to antigens (also named *apoptotic death*) is absent in most lymphoid malignancies, with the notable exception of Burkitt's lymphoma. Follicular center cell lymphomas account for approximately 30% of all NHLs and are particularly prevalent in the elderly. They frequently present with generalized adenopathy and paratrabecular marrow involvement. Despite early dissemination, these "low-grade" lymphomas respond quite well to chemotherapy for several years before their eventual vindictive transformation to more aggressive histology.

Diffuse large cell lymphomas (diffuse histiocytic lymphomas [DHLs]) are among the commonest NHLs. They are characterized by B cell centroblastic proliferations, bulky, often extranodal, tumors, and intermediate-grade progression. The diffuse cytology of these gross tumors (**Figure 49-4,** ×1,260) features disorderly sheets of large centroblasts, admixed with a minor population of small, dark, flattened, or cleaved centrocytes. The predominant centroblasts have big (sometimes huge), ovoid, clear nuclei with 1 or more distinctive nucleoli, which are often attached to the thickened nuclear membrane. Most noncleaved cells have moderate amounts of eosinophilic cytoplasm, which often interlocks with that of neighboring cells, creating a pattern of patchy cohesion. Some large cells are notched, lobated, or cleaved, and cells with deeply folded nuclei and prominent central nucleoli may resemble RS cells. The finding of only a single mitotic figure in this field (lower right) might be interpreted as a favorable prognostic sign. Accurate evaluation of mitotic activity depends on expeditious fixation of biopsy material, however, for cycling cells kept waiting en route to the pathology lab can slip through mitosis unnoticed. The cells of this diffuse lymphoma are large because a high percentage are in active cell cycle. This makes them highly vulnerable to cycle-dependent chemotherapeutic agents. The paradoxical and happy consequence is that in over half of patients these aggressive lymphomas can be cured.

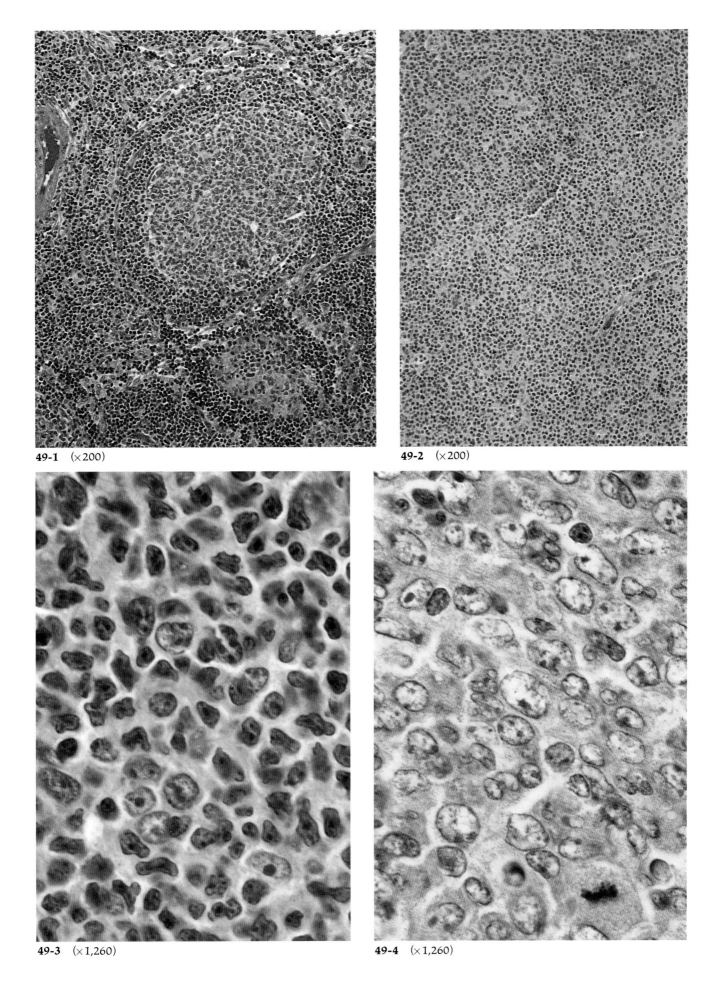

49-1 (×200)

49-2 (×200)

49-3 (×1,260)

49-4 (×1,260)

Figure 50. High-Grade Non-Hodgkin's Lymphomas. (H&E–stained sections).

Several histologically distinctive nodal neoplasms are classified as high-grade non-Hodgkin's lymphomas because of their explosive growth and deadly course. Collectively, high-grade NHLs account for 15 to 20% of all lymphomas, with the incidence of several kinds rising sharply in this era of immunosuppression by chemotherapy, radiotherapy, and HIV infection. The most common of these malign processes are the large cell immunoblastic lymphomas, most of which are of B cell origin, the rest being high-grade T cell cancers.

B immunoblastic sarcoma (B-IBS), an extremely aggressive lyphoma of plasma cell precursors (immunoblasts), is a nemesis of the immunosuppressed, including victims of AIDS. The picturesque plasmacytoid tumor cells possess startling pleomorphism (**Figure 50-1**, ×1,260). The cytoplasm is densely eosinophilic (and pyroninophilic), contains dark blotchy inclusions, and has cracking artifacts caused by condensation of immunoglobulin deposits. Nuclei are blastlike, with prominent, often single, centroidal nuclei. The malignant population includes bizarre multilobated and multinucleated giant forms that may bear an eerie resemblance to Reed-Sternberg (RS) cells. The binucleate RS mimic at the top of this figure can be distinguished from the real thing by the dense eosinophilia of the cytoplasm, the dark purple (not red) nucleoli, and the accompanying troupe of plasmacytoid variants. In Hodgkin's disease, RS cells stand out starkly against a surrounding lymphoid population of comparative midgets; in B-IBS, a continuum exists extending from giant forms to small immunoblasts, some of which contain mitotic figures (upper right). To avoid misidentification, it is prudent to set aside frozen sections for subsequent cell marker studies. The diagnosis of B-IBS can be established by use of B cell markers for monoclonal sIg, cIg, and heavy (H) and light (L) chains.

T immunoblastic sarcoma (T-IBS), a tumor of nodal T cell origin, is apt to invade the mediastinum, lungs, and pleura at the outset—unlike B-IBS, which commonly presents in the central nervous system. T immunoblasts have large water-clear nuclei containing 1 or more small, dark, red-purple nucleoli (**Figure 50-2**, ×1,260). The pale vesicular nuclei are surrounded by a thin rim of cytoplasm that is retracted by shrinkage artifact to create a characteristic corona or *clear zone*. In the *polymorphic variant of T-IBS* shown here, the large clear cells are admixed with numerous small lymphocytes having dark, knobby, twisted, irregular nuclei characteristic of T lymphocytes. Occasionally B-IBS cytology may simulate the clear cell cytology of T-IBS, a possibility that can be explored by rounding up the usual B cell marker suspects. As befits tumor cells, T cell marker studies are sometimes foiled by antigenic aberrations or omissions, so that a full panel of markers should be used: this normally includes antibodies to CD2, CD4, CD8, CD7, and CD3. Correct phenotyping is not particularly vital for prognosis but is of potential value should T cell purging of an autologous marrow transplant be contemplated.

Lymphoblastic lymphoma is a solid state counterpart to T cell ALL, similarly affecting young males and presenting as an anterior mediastinal mass that disseminates rapidly to marrow and brain. The medium size tumor cells are notable for their *convoluted nuclei*, speckled chromatin, thick nuclear membranes, and scant cytoplasm. The degree of cell crowding and nuclear deformation is unrivalled among other lymphomas (**Figure 50-3**, ×1,260). Nuclear membranes possess multiple deep folds, creases, and grooves, creating busy nuclear convolutions and lobulations. The histology simulates a tray of shelled pecans. Crowds of wrinkled lymphoblasts are relieved only by mitotic figures and occasional tingible body macrophages. Cytology of lymphoblastic lymphoma differs from that of the more merciful and prevalent small cleaved cell lymphoma in that most nuclei have complex creases rather than a single plane of cleavage, and the mitotic rate is much higher, forecasting speedier progression.

Diffuse small noncleaved cell lymphomas comprise a group of very high-grade tumors of children or young adults. This category includes *Burkitt's lymphoma* endemic to the tropics, the sporadic American version known as *Burkitt's-like lymphoma*, and a fast-growing *undifferentiated lymphoma*, which often emerges as a terminal consequence of HIV infection. Burkitt's lymphomas, endemic or sporadic, are composed of compact masses of medium size lymphocytes whose round nuclei abut or overlap, causing the cytoplasm of neighboring cells to merge. Chromatin is dispersed in a stippled or polka-dot pattern overlaid by 1 to 3 bold nucleoli (**Figure 50-4**, ×800). Mitotic figures abound, signifying a high birth (and death) rate of tumor cells. The doubling times of these B cell tumors are often as brief as 24 to 48 hours, making Burkitt's and Burkitt's-like lymphomas the fastest growing of human cancers. The high associated cell death rate attracts scavenging macrophages, and the interspersion of these large pale "histiocytes" (upper left), set off against the crammed multitudes of tumor cells, is responsible for the celebrated *starry sky* effect. The lymphoma cells look quite different in Wright-Giemsa stained imprint preparations, in which the unshrunk cytoplasm stands out, deeply basophilic and filled with pearly vacuoles. Burkitt's lymphoma cells have the phenotype of mature B cells (sIg$^+$, CD20$^+$), and both the endemic and sporadic tumors are associated with translocations that juxtapose the *c-myc* oncogene of chromosome 8 and Ig gene loci. The most common rearrangement is the famed 8;14 translocation.

True histiocytic lymphoma (**Figure 50-5**, ×1,260) is an uncommon tumor of macrophage derivation, characterized by diffuse infiltration, large cells with copious eosinophilic cytoplasm, corpulent nuclei, and 1 to 3 irregular nucleoli. The folded nuclei and heavy nuclear membranes are lineaments of monocyte ancestry, as can be verified by surface markers, by demonstrating nonspecific esterase, and by identifying characteristic degradative enzymes, including α_1-antitrypsin, α_1-antichymotrypsin, and lysozyme. Frequent mitoses and scattered pyknotic debris attest to high birth and death rates.

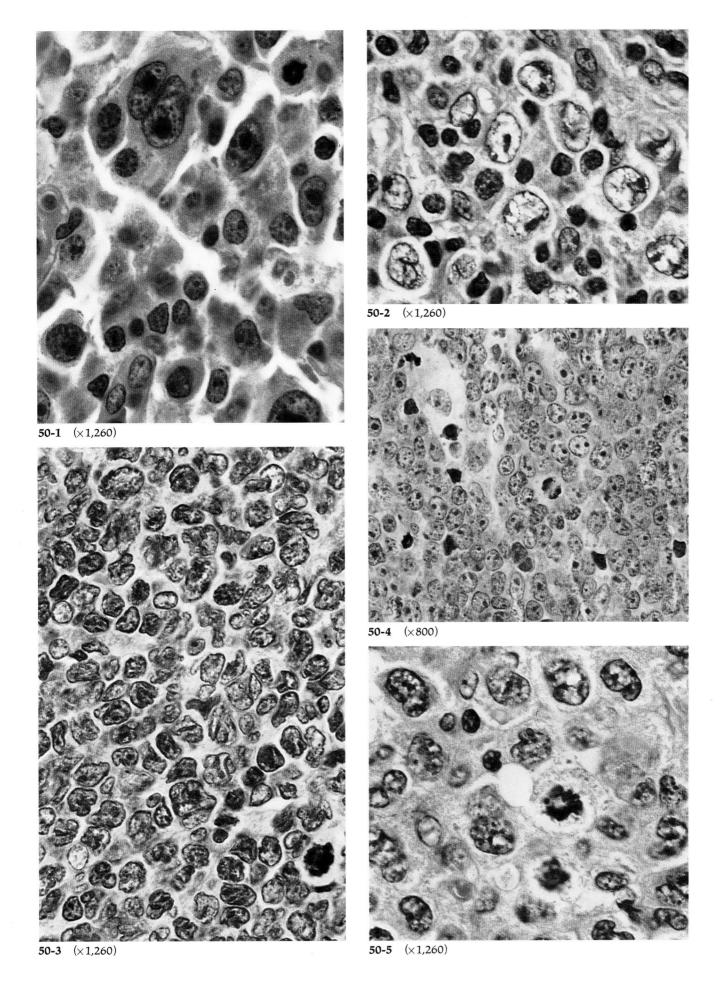

50-1 (×1,260)

50-2 (×1,260)

50-3 (×1,260)

50-4 (×800)

50-5 (×1,260)

Figure 51. Sézary Cells and Other Lymphoma Cells in Blood. Lymphoma Cell Leukemias.

The triptych of cells at the top of this page is meant as a treasury of cells named for Sézary. The 3 cell portraits presented in **Figures 51-1, 51-2,** and **51-3** (all ×2,000) typify these renowned cells as they appear in the course of *cutaneous T cell lymphomas* (CTCLs). *Sézary cells* range from slightly enlarged to twice the size of normal T cells, the larger ones (cellules monstreuses) possessing dark, metachromatic, tetraploid nuclei. The tumor cells are heterogeneous and vary in their dimensions and proportions from one patient to the next. The large cell variants often have deeply infolded nuclei that may be described as cerebriform (**Figure 51-1**) or convoluted (**Figure 51-2**). In the small cell variants, convolutions may be so tortured that nuclei resemble mulberries. Nuclear convolutions in both large and small Sézary cells are baroque in their intricacy when viewed by transmission electron microscopy. The scant to moderate amount of blue-gray cytoplasm often contains 1 or 2 dozen clear vacuoles arranged like a strand of pearls (**Figure 51-3**). A single strand of these PAS-positive vesicles hugging the nuclear perimeter bears a fanciful likeness to a choker necklace.

CTCL is an insidious, disfiguring disorder with protean manifestations once grouped separately under the venerable terms, *mycosis fungoides* and *Sézary syndrome.* CTCL originates in lymph nodes as a low-grade malignancy of T4 cells. The mutant lymphocytes possess a singular epidermotropism that causes them to home in on the upper dermis and epidermis. Tumor cells thrive in skin colonies known as *Pautrier's abscesses,* from which they spread through a staged evolution to cause erythroderma, unsightly plaques, and, eventually, appalling conglomerations of cutaneous and nodal tumors. Sézary cells can be identified in the blood of over half of patients during the plaque phase of disease, and, in patients with systemic infiltration and lymphoid tumors, frank Sézary-cell leukemias may ensue, with white counts reaching 100,000/µl. Diagnosis rests on skin biopsy and discovery in blood smears of lymphocytes having a cerebriform nucleus and a diameter exceeding 14 µm. Identification of this degrading and demoralizing disorder is imperative, for both cutaneous and systemic therapies are available.

Sensitive flow cytometric methods combined with marker studies such as kappa/lambda analysis indicate that more than 80% of patients presenting with active non-Hodgkin's lymphoma have monoclonal populations of tumor cells in the circulation. Even in low-grade follicular lymphomas, clonal B cells persist in the bloodstream throughout therapy-induced remission, explaining the perverse penchant for later relapse. The morphology of circulating lymphoma cells reflects the histologic type of the tumor, but structural details are more open to view in Wright-Giemsa stained smears than in H&E–stained reactions. The coloring is incomparably brighter, subtler, and more luminous. The panoptic pulchritude of blood lymphocytes in the *leukemic phase of Burkitt's lymphoma* (**Figure 51-4,** ×2,000) attests to the triumph of spread smears over tissue artifacts. Unlike the bland, lackluster look of Burkitt's lymphoma cells in H&E–stained sections (see **Figure 50-4**), the same tumor cells in circulation bloom with the vivid coloration of transformed B cells. These leukemic cells are identical to those of the L3 type of acute lymphatic leukemia occurring de novo (see **Figure 42-3**). The abundant cytoplasm of these 2 representative cells is darkly basophilic, especially along the margins, which may hug the contours of neighboring red cells. In many cells, as exemplified on the left, the cytoplasm is pierced by clear vacuoles, and the oblong or slightly folded violet nuclei contain up to 5 vague nucleoli.

Occurrence of lymphoma cell leukemia in patients with *diffuse large cell lymphoma* is an ominous turn, predictive of short survival. The great size of these robust cells (about 30 µm across) is more imposing in blood smears (**Figure 51-5,** ×1,260) than in fixed sections, where shrinkage artifact reduces cell dimensions by nearly half. Note the opaque, curdled, plasmacytoid cytoplasm and several smudged nucleoli in the eccentric nucleus. More than 20% of *follicular small cleaved cell lymphomas* convert to a leukemic phase and are responsible for the majority of "chronic" lymphoma cell leukemias. The cleaved cells and angular forms seen in sections become spread out and reveal a multiplicity of complex cleavage patterns when tumor cells enter the blood and wind up on a glass slide or coverslip (**Figure 51-6,** ×1,260). Note the bold single nucleolus in some of these multilobular nuclei. Enormous centroidal nucleoli are the medallions of *B immunoblastic sarcoma* cells (**Figure 51-7,** ×1,260) when these become bloodborne during terminal dissemination. The malign purport of these invasive cells can be recognized from their cycloptic glare.

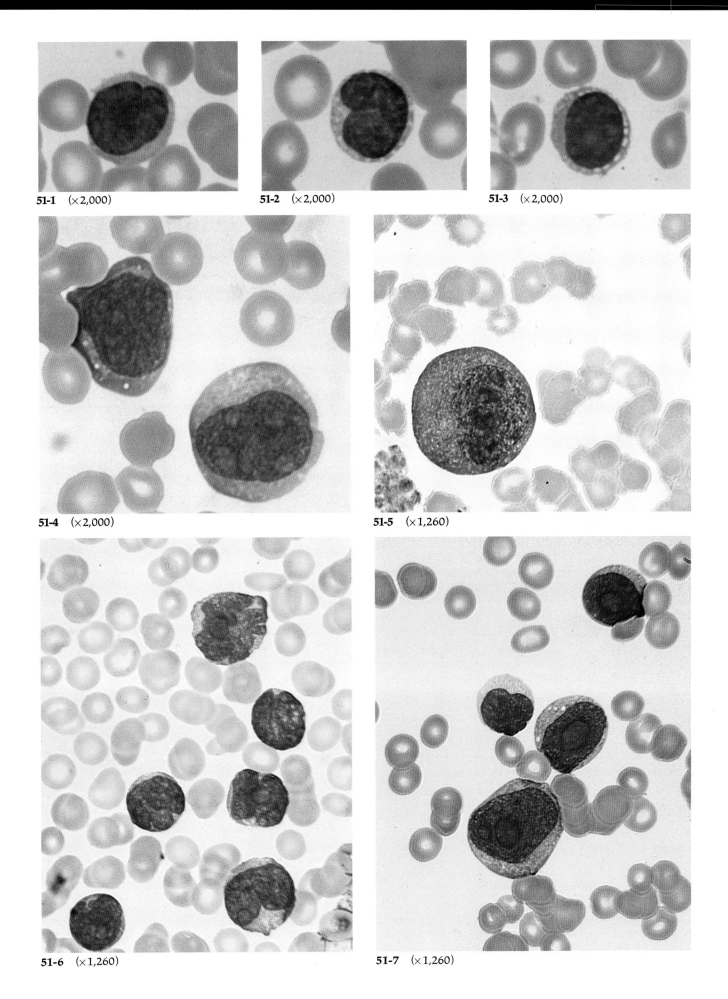

51-1 (×2,000)

51-2 (×2,000)

51-3 (×2,000)

51-4 (×2,000)

51-5 (×1,260)

51-6 (×1,260)

51-7 (×1,260)

Bibliography

Hodgkin's Disease

Fuller LM et al, Eds: Hodgkin's Disease and Non-Hodgkin's Lymphomas in Adults and Children. New York, Raven Press, 1988

Garratty G et al: Autoimmune hemolytic anemia in Hodgkin's disease associated with and anti-I^T. Transfusion 14 : 226, 1974

Glaser SL: Recent incidence and secular trends in Hodgkin's disease and its histologic subtypes. J Chronic Dis 39 : 789, 1986

Gutensohn NM: Social class and age at diagnosis of Hodgkin's disease: new epidemiologic evidence for the "two-disease hypothesis." Cancer Treat Rep 66 : 689, 1982

Hagemeister FB: Prognostic factors in decision-making in the clinical management of Hodgkin's disease. Hematol Oncol 6 : 257, 1988

Halie MR: Observations on abnormal cells in the peripheral blood and spleen in Hodgkin's disease. Br Med J 2 : 609, 1972

Hancock BW et al: Lymphopenia. A bad prognostic factor in Hodgkin's disease. Scand J Haematol 29 : 193, 1982

Hoppe RT: The contemporary management of Hodgkin disease. Radiology 169 : 297, 1988

Hunter JD et al: Autoimmune neutropenia in Hodgkin's disease. Arch Intern Med 142 : 386, 1982

Jandl JH: Chapt 27, in Blood: Textbook of Hematology. Boston, Little, Brown and Company, 1987

Kaplan HS: Hodgkin's Disease, 2nd ed. Cambridge, Harvard University Press, 1980

Levine AM et al: Positive Coombs test in Hodgkin's disease: significance and implications. Blood 55 : 607, 1980

MacLennan KA et al: The pretreatment peripheral blood lymphocyte count in 1100 patients with Hodgkin's disease: the prognostic signficance and the relationship to the presence of systemic symptoms. Clin Oncol 7 : 333, 1981

Weiss LM et al: Detection of Epstein-Barr viral genomes in Reed-Sternberg cells of Hodgkin's disease. N Engl J Med 320 : 502, 1989

Weitberg AB and Harmon DC: Autoimmune neutropenia, hemolytic anemia, and reticulocytopenia in Hodgkin's disease. Ann Intern Med 100 : 702, 1984

Non-Hodgkin's Lymphomas

Abboud SL et al: Well-differentiated lymphocytic lymphoma with peripheral blood involvement, osteolytic bone lesions, and hypercalcemia. A case report and review of the literature. Cancer 56 : 2508, 1985

Armitage JO et al: Peripheral T-cell lymphoma. Cancer 63 : 158, 1989

Broder S and Bunn PA Jr: Cutaneous T-cell lymphoma. Semin Oncol 7 : 310, 1980

Buzzanga J et al: Lymph node histopathology in Sezary syndrome. J Am Acad Dermatol 11 : 880, 1984

Canellos GP: Section 12, Subsection XI. Malignant lymphomas, in Scientific American Medicine, Rubenstein E and Federman DD, Eds. New York, Scientific American, Inc, 1988

Cohen LF et al: Acute tumor lysis syndrome. A review of 37 patients with Burkitt's lymphoma. Am J Med 68 : 486, 1980

Come SE et al: Non-Hodgkin's lymphomas in leukemic phase: clinicopathologic correlations. Am J Med 69 : 667, 1980

Donner LR et al: Angiocentric immunoproliferative lesion (lymphomatoid granulomatosis). Cancer 65 : 249, 1990

Duggan MJ et al: Mantle zone lymphoma. A clinicopathological study of 22 cases. Cancer 66 : 522, 1990

Eddy JL et al: Cutaneous T-cell lymphoma. Am J Nursing 84 : 202, 1984

Fauci A et al: Lymphomatoid granulomatosis. Prospective clinical and therapeutic experience over 10 years. N Engl J Med 306 : 68, 1982

Flandrin G et al: Acute leukemia with Burkitt's tumor cells: A study of six cases with special reference to lymphocyte surface markers. Blood 45 : 183, 1975

Fuller LM et al, Eds: Hodgkin's Disease and Non-Hodgkin's Lymphomas in Adults and Children. New York, Raven Press, 1988

Green TL and Eversole LR: Oral lymphomas in HIV-infected patients: association with Epstein-Barr virus DNA. Oral Surg Oral Med Oral Pathol 67 : 437, 1989

Greer JP et al: Peripheral T-cell lymphoma: a clinicopathologic study of 42 cases. J Clin Oncol 2 : 788, 1984

Hernandez JA and Sheehan WW: Lymphomas of the mucosa-associated lymphoid tissue. Signet ring cell lymphomas presenting in mucosal lymphoid organs. Cancer 55 : 592, 1985

Hu E et al: Diagnosis of B cell lymphoma by analysis of immunoglobulin gene rearrangements in biopsy specimens obtained by fine needle aspiration. J Clin Oncol 4 : 278, 1986

Iwahara K and Hashimoto K: T-cell subsets and nuclear contour index of skin-infiltrating T-cells in cutaneous T-cell lymphoma. Cancer 54 : 440, 1984

Jaffe ES et al: Predictability of immunologic phenotype by morphologic criteria in diffuse aggressive non-Hodgkin's lymphomas. Am J Clin Pathol 77 : 46, 1982

Jaffe ES et al: Malignant lymphoma and erythrophagocytosis simulating malignant histiocytosis. Am J Med 75 : 741, 1983

Jaffe ES: Chapt 9, in Atlas of Blood Cells: Function and Pathology, vol. 1, Zucker-Franklin D et al, Eds. Milan, Edi. Ermes s.r.l., 1988

Jambrosic J et al: Lymphomatoid granulomatosis. J Am Acad Dermatol 17 : 621, 1987

Jandl JH: Chapt 28, in Blood: Textbook of Hematology. Boston, Little, Brown and Company, 1987

Kearns DB et al: Burkitt's lymphoma. Int J Pediatr Otorhinolaryngol 12 : 73, 1986

Knowles DM et al: Clinicopathologic, immunophenotypic, and molecular genetic analysis of AIDS-associated lymphoid neoplasia. Clinical and biologic implications. Pathol Annu 23(part 2) : 33, 1988

Knowles DM et al: Molecular genetic analysis of three AIDS-associated neoplasms of uncertain lineage demonstrates their B-cell derivation and the possible pathogenetic role of the Epstein-Barr virus. Blood 73 : 792, 1989

Krueger GRF et al: A New Working Formulation of non-Hodgkin's lymphomas. A retrospective study of the new NCI classification proposal in comparison to the Rappaport and Kiel classifications. Cancer 52 : 833, 1983

Levine AM et al: Small noncleaved follicular center cell (FCC) lymphoma: Burkitt and non-Burkitt variants in the United States. I. Clinical features. Cancer 52 : 1073, 1983

Lichtenstein A et al: Immunoblastic sarcoma: a clinical description. Cancer 43 : 343, 1979

Ligler FS et al: Detection of tumor cells in the peripheral blood of nonleukemic patients with B-cell lymphoma: analysis of "clonal excess." Blood 55 : 792, 1980

Lindh J et al: Monoclonal B cells in peripheral blood in non-Hodgkin's lymphoma. Correlation with clinical features and DNA content. Scand J Haematol 32 : 5, 1984

Lipford EH Jr et al: Angiocentric immunoproliferative lesions: a clinicopathologic spectrum of post-thymic T-cell proliferations. Blood 72 : 1674, 1988

Long JC et al : Terminal deoxynucleotidyl transferase positive lymphoblastic lymphoma: a study of 15 cases. Cancer 44 : 2127, 1979

Magrath IT, Ed: The Non-Hodgkin's Lymphomas. Baltimore, Williams & Wilkins, 1990

Mathe G et al: Leukemic conversion of non-Hodgkin's lymphomata. Br J Cancer 32(Suppl 2) : 96, 1975

Michel RP et al: Immunoblastic lymphosarcoma: a light, immunofluorescence, and electron microscopic study. Cancer 43 : 224, 1979

Miliauskas JR et al: Undifferentiated non-Hodgkin's lymphomas (Burkitt's and non-Burkitt's types): the relevance of making this histologic distinction. Cancer 50 : 2115, 1982

Minerbrook M et al: Burkitt's leukemia: a re-evaluation. Cancer 49 : 1444, 1982

Mintzer DM and Hauptman SP: Lymphosarcoma cell leukemia and other non-Hodgkin's lymphomas in leukemic phase. Am J Med 75 : 110, 1983

Morra E et al: Leukemic phase of non-Hodgkin's lymphomas, hematological features and prognostic significance. Haematologica 69 : 15, 1984

Nathwani BN et al: Lymphoblastic lymphoma: a clinicopathologic study of 95 patients. Cancer 48 : 2347, 1981

Newell GR et al: Incidence of lymphoma in the US classified by the Working Formulation. Cancer 59 : 857, 1987

Ngan B-Y et al: Detection of chromosomal translocation t(14;18) within the minor cluster region of bcl-2 by polymerase chain reaction and direct genomic sequencing of the enzymatically amplified DNA in follicular lymphomas. Blood 73 : 1759, 1989

Patton LL et al: American Burkitt's lymphoma: a 10-year review and case study. Oral Surg Oral Med Oral Pathol 69 : 307, 1990

Ralfkiaer E et al: Sezary syndrome: phenotypic and functional characterization of the neoplastic cells. Scand J Haematol 34 : 385, 1985

Robb-Smith AHT and Taylor CR: Lymph Node Biopsy: a Diagnostic Atlas. New York, Oxford University Press, 1981

Said JW and Pinkus GS: Immunologic characterization and ultrastructural correlations for 125 cases of B- and T-cell leukemias: studies of chronic and acute lymphocytic, pro-lymphocytic, lymphosarcoma cell and hairy cell leukemia, Sezary's syndrome, and other lymphoid leukemias. Cancer 48 : 2630, 1981

Smith BR et al: Circulating monoclonal B-lymphocytes in non-Hodgkin's lymphoma. N Engl J Med 311 : 1476, 1984

Stuart AE et al, Eds: Chapt 1, in Lymphomas Other Than Hodgkin's Disease. Oxford, Oxford University Press, 1981

Tashiro K et al: Clinicopathological study of Ki-1-positive lymphomas. Pathol Res Pract 185 : 461, 1989

Thomas P et al: True histiocytic lymphoma: an immunohistochemical and ultrastructural study of two cases. Am J Clin Pathol 81 : 243, 1984

Tindle BH: Malignant lymphomas. Am J Pathol 116 : 115, 1984

Van der Loo EM et al: The prognostic value of membrane markers and morphometric characteristics of lymphoid cells in blood and lymph nodes from patients with mycosis fungoides. Cancer 48 : 738, 1981

van der Putte SCJ et al: Cutaneous T-cell lymphoma, multilobated type. Histopathology 6 : 35, 1982

van der Putte SCJ et al: Cutaneous T-cell lymphoma, multilobated type, expressing membrane differentiation antigens of precursor T-lymphocytes. Br J Dermatol 107 : 293, 1982

van der Valk P et al: Malignant lymphoma of true histiocytic origin: histiocytic sarcoma. A morphological, ultrastructural, immunological, cytochemical and clinical study of 10 cases. Virchows Arch [A] 391 : 249, 1981

Weinberg DS and Pinkus GS: Non-Hodgkin's lymphoma of large multilobated cell type. A clinicopathologic study of ten cases. Am J Clin Pathol 76 : 190, 1981

Winkler CF and Bunn PA Jr: Cutaneous T-cell lymphoma: a review. CRC Crit Rev Oncol Hematol 1 : 49, 1983

Yamada Y et al: T lymphomas associated with human T-cell leukemia-lymphoma virus may show phenotypic and functional differences from adult T-cell leukemias. Clin Immunol Immunopathol 36 : 306, 1985

Yamaguchi K et al: Lymphoma type adult T-cell leukemia—a clinicopathologic study of HTLV related T-cell type malignant lymphoma. Hematol Oncol 4 : 59, 1986

Ziegler JL: Burkitt's lymphoma. N Engl J Med 305 : 735, 1981

VII. Lymphoproliferative
Reactions

Figure 52. Infectious Mononucleosis. Atypical Lymphocytes.

Infectious mononucleosis is an acute viral infection characterized by fever, pharyngitis, lymphadenopathy, splenomegaly, and an outpouring into the bloodstream of picturesque populations of *variant* or *atypical lymphocytes*. The disease is caused by a human herpesvirus known as *Epstein-Barr virus* (EBV), which binds to C3d (CR2) receptors on the surfaces of B cells in lymphoid tissue of the tonsils and Waldeyer's ring. Occupancy of these receptors transforms B cells, immortalizes them, and drives them to disseminate throughout the circulation. The flaunting of obnoxious viral antigens by infected B cells is first protested by natural killer cells, constitutive defenders against viruses being smuggled in by antigen-presenting B cells. Battle-scarred, degranulated NK cells (large granular lymphocytes) become the first cytologic emblem of infection (**Figure 52-1,** ×2,000). These valiant elements of the first wave of atypical lymphocytes are large pale cells, with oblong or bean-shaped nuclei and vacuolated cytoplasm. Degranulated NK cells, once cataloged as Downey type I cells, resemble Sézary cells in their size, hyperchromatic nuclei, and circumferential beaded strings of vacuoles. As they are engaged on the ramparts of the tonsils, the first full fury of the outraged T cell network is unleashed. Within 1 week of onset, armies of transformed T cells begin to storm all infected outposts and to search out and destroy collaborating B cells on sight. The ranks of this second and larger wave of atypical lymphocytes are filled by cytolytic and suppressor T8 cells. Newly transformed cytolytic T cells are large (18 to 25 μm across), hyperdiploid, and blastlike, with copious darkly basophilic cytoplasm and youthful nuclei containing impressive nucleoli (**Figure 52-2,** ×2,000).

Transformed T8 cells can resemble ALL lymphoblasts and may show block positivity on PAS staining. When these malevolent-looking young lymphocytes are numerous, it is advisable to monitor differential counts to be assured that the blastlike cells are transients. Cytolytic and suppressor T cells account for the bulk of atypical lymphocytes that are so dramatic a feature of infectious mononucleosis during the second, third, and fourth weeks of illness. Warlike in demeanor as well as appearance, cytolytic T cells pounce on and lyse B cells bearing EBV antigens (lymphocyte-detected membrane antigens, or LYDMA). This assault eliminates all infected B cells from circulation and confines immortalized forms to small nodal sanctuaries, from which they may escape only during immunosuppression. A third population of T cells that emerges during the immune response to EBV infection is composed of large ameboid cells with voluminous pale blue cytoplasm, which is darkened and artfully furled ("skirted") at the margins (**Figure 52-3,** ×2,000). The curious propensity of skirted lymphocytes to embrace or adhere to the rounded contours of neighboring red cells, sometimes promiscuously, has inevitably earned them the sobriquet of "kissing cells." In producing kissing cells, nature both imitates art and provides a suggestive clue to pathogenesis. Infectious mononucleosis is only weakly contagious in young adults. For a susceptible adult to be infected by a healthy carrier requires prolonged and impassioned osculation, with bulk exchange of buccal fluids. The morphologic diversity and magnitude of lymphocyte responses to EBV products, while not pathognomonic, are extraordinary because of the multiplicity of T cell and NK cell subsets brought into play.

EBV infection elicits a predictable sequence of antibodies to the virus itself and to altered components of the host's B cells. None of the EBV-specific antigens is responsible for evoking the mysterious *heterophil antibody* of the Paul-Bunnell type, antibody that plays no known role in defense but serves as a valued diagnostic indicator. Slide tests (such as Monospot) employing formalinized horse red cells should be performed with disposable equipment and glove precautions to minimize exposure to hepatitis B and HIV.

Many self-limited infections or allergic reactions may cause *heterophil-negative mononucleosis syndromes* in which blood morphology simulates that of infectious mononucleosis. Comparably atypical lymphocytes may appear as a particularly puzzling feature of *cytomegalovirus* (CMV) infection, the common contagions of childhood, infectious hepatitis, and toxoplasmosis. Infection by CMV and many other systemic viruses may elicit "atypical" T cell and NK cell responses indistinguishable from those in infectious mononucleosis (**Figure 52-5,** ×2,000). This patient also had the misfortune of experiencing renal shutdown, which accounts for the numerous uremic burr cells. During hypersensitivity reactions to antigens or drugs, transformed T cells may be joined by activated B cells displaying plasmacytoid features (**Figure 52-4,** ×2,000). These 2 lymphocytes from a patient with serum sickness have the opaque blue-gray cytoplasm and slightly eccentric mature nuclei of secretory B cells, or plymphs. The mixed cellular responses to antigenic drugs are shown in extended detail in **Figure 53.**

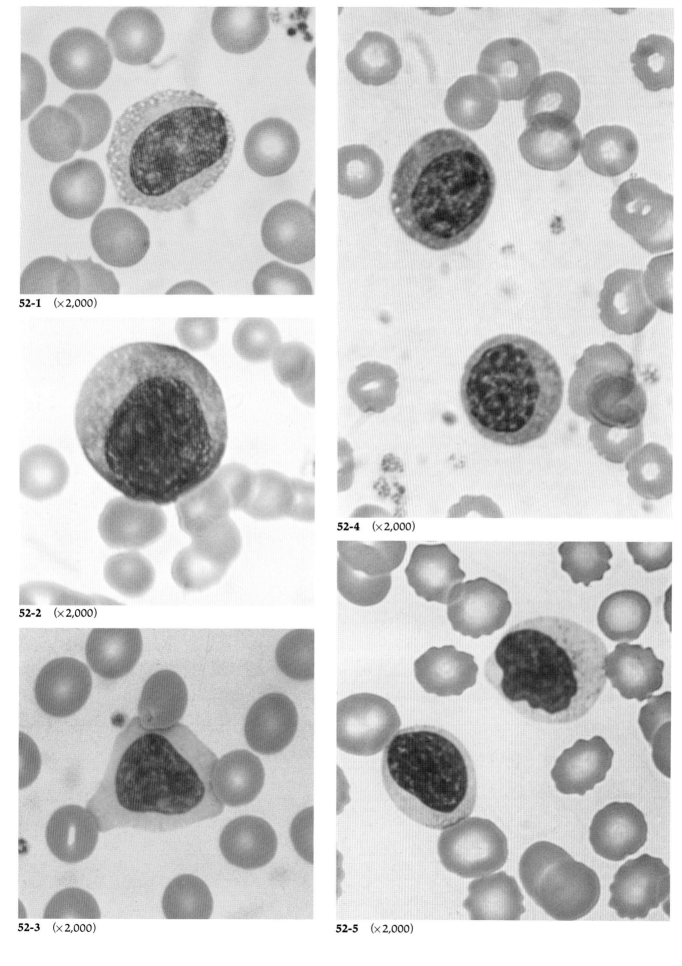

52-1 (×2,000)

52-2 (×2,000)

52-3 (×2,000)

52-4 (×2,000)

52-5 (×2,000)

Figure 53. Drug-induced Reactions

Figures 53-1 through **53-5** (all ×1,260 except **Figure 53-3,** ×2,000) present a pastiche of portraits of atypical lymphocytes caused by hypersensitivity reactions to medications. Drug-induced reactions have become the commonest cause of atypical lymphocytosis. Recognition of this connection and of the morphologic patterns involved serves not only to warn of adverse reactions requiring discontinuance of offending medications but spares the perils and expense of contingent diagnostic meddling. **Figure 53-1** portrays the worrisome morphology observed in a patient experiencing a vigorous hypersensitivity reaction to an antirheumatic nostrum. Apart from the 2 mutilated eosinophils on the right, all nucleated cells are lymphocytes. Despite shrinkage artifacts in this excessively thick smear, several aberrations are evident. The large glowering lymphocyte near the top has a threatening countenance, but its deeply basophilic cytoplasm and well-condensed nuclear chromatin indicate that this is not a blast. The basophilia and hyperdiploid nuclear lobulation suggest that this lymphocyte has recently undergone reactive transformation. All of the smaller lymphocytes in this field also possess deep blue cytoplasm, and all nuclei are tightly lobulated, indented, or grooved, indicating that this is a collection of young T cells. A lymphocyte at the center has a perinuclear collar of pearly vacuoles; except for its small size, this could be mistaken for a Sézary cell.

Many drug-induced immunologic reactions elicit formidable lymphoproliferative responses that may surpass infectious mononucleosis in their intimation of menace. After a transient period of leukopenia, large, irregular, deeply basophilic forms appear that may include robust blastoid lymphocytes possessing huge and sometimes multiple nucleoli (**Figures 53-2** and **53-3**). Some reassurance is supplied by the mixed company these blasts keep—assorted "typical atypical" lymphocytes, plasma cells, plymphs, and eosinophils (**Figures 53-2** and **53-4**). There is no denying the neoplastic look of the big blasts shown in **Figures 53-3** and **53-5,** which have all the features of malignant lymphoblasts. Despite assurance from the company-kept rule, diagnostic confidence comes only when these ominous things disappear. As hypersensitivity reactions progress, a rogue's gallery of atypical lymphocytes may come and go. Absent only are the big blue-margined ameboid forms that grace the morphology of infectious mononucleosis. Included among the evanescent cast of characters that may parade by during acute immune reactions are simulators of Sézary cells, hairy cells, lymphomalike cleaved cells, and other forms that, if persistent, would ordinarily serve as marker cells for lymphocytic malignancies. Drug reactions are imitations of the venerable immunologic response to "foreign" (heterologous) protein known as *serum sickness*. During this violent reaction, as occurs following infusion of horse antithymocyte globulin, the same colorful succession of atypical lymphocytes, plasma cells, and eosinophils occurs.

As noted in **Figure 52,** many self-limited infections can cause heterophil-negative mononucleosis syndromes that must be differentiated from the drug-induced and serum sickness reactions described above. Among the infectious agents responsible are rubella, adenovirus, *Toxoplasma gondii*, hepatitis viruses, and CMV. In recent years CMV infection has outstripped the other causes of this syndrome because of the cumulative numbers of patients rendered vulnerable to this ubiquitous virus by immunosuppressive disease (AIDS) or cytotoxic therapy. Initially referred to as *posttransfusion syndrome*, CMV infection is a hazard for patients who are massively transfused or are recipients of organ transplants. Infection is marked by the same weird assortment of atypical lymphocytes found in infectious mononucleosis.

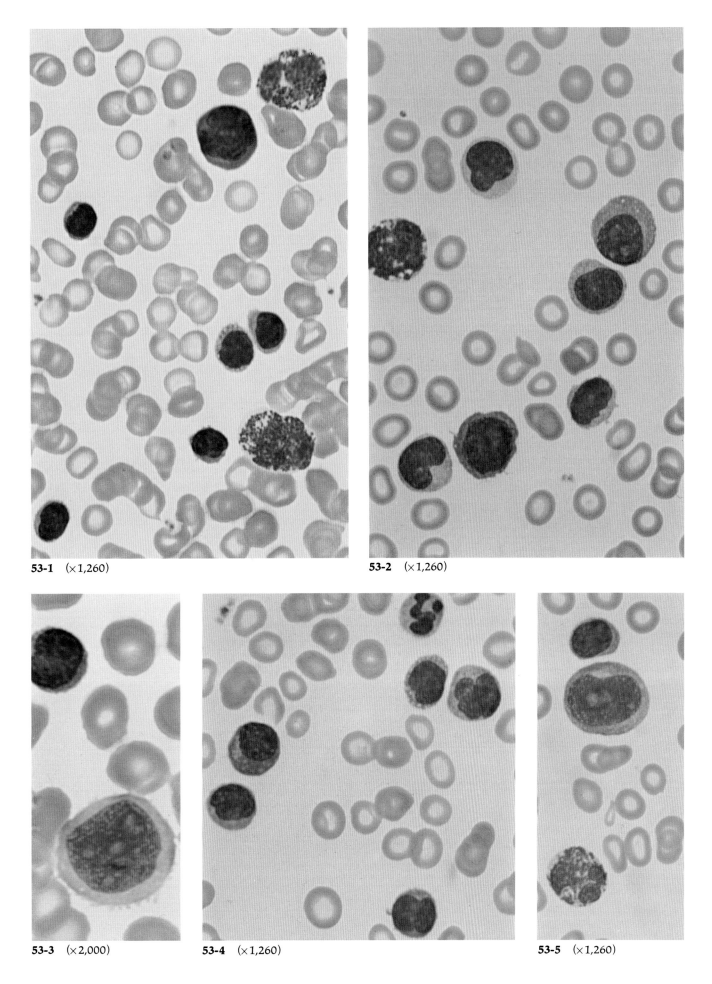

53-1　(×1,260)

53-2　(×1,260)

53-3　(×2,000)

53-4　(×1,260)

53-5　(×1,260)

Bibliography

Betts RF: Syndrome of cytomegalovirus infection. Adv Intern Med 26 : 447, 1980

Bierer BE et al:T-cell activation: the T-cell erythrocyte receptor (CD2) and sialophorin (CD42). Immunol Allergy Clin North Am 8 : 51, 1988

Bishop CJ et al: T lymphocytes in infectious mononucleosis. II. Response in vitro to interleukin-2 and establishment of T cell lines. Clin Exp Immunol 60 : 70, 1985

Burdette S and Schwartz RS: Idiotypes and idiotypic networks. N Engl J Med 317 : 219, 1987

Cleary ML and Sklar J: Lymphoproliferative disorders in cardiac transplant recipients are multiclonal lymphomas. Lancet 1 : 489, 1984

Cooper MD: B lymphocytes. Normal development and function. N Engl J Med 317 : 1452, 1987

Epstein MA and Achong BG: Pathogenesis of infectious mononucleosis. Lancet 2 : 1270, 1977

Fiala M et al: Infectious mononucleosis and mononucleosis syndromes. West J Med 126 : 445, 1977

Finch SC: Chapt 2, in Infectious Mononucleosis, Carter RL and Penman HG, Eds. Oxford, Blackwell Scientific Publications, 1969

Gilliland BC: Serum sickness and immune complexes. N Engl J Med 311 : 1435, 1984

Grossi CE et al: Chapt 9, in Atlas of Blood Cells: Function and Pathology. Zucker-Franklin D et al, Eds. Milan, Edi. Ermes s.r.l., 1988

Harrington DS et al: Epstein-Barr virus–associated lymphoproliferative lesions. Clin Lab Med 8 : 97, 1988

Hoagland RJ: Infectious Mononucleosis. New York, Grune & Stratton, Inc, 1967

Horwitz CA et al: Clinical and laboratory evaluation of elderly patients with heterophil-antibody positive infectious mononucleosis. Report of seven patients, ages 40 to 78. Am J Med 61 : 333, 1976

Horwitz CA et al: Heterophil-negative infectious mononucleosis. Am J Med 63 : 947, 1977

Jaffe E, Ed: Surgical Pathology of the Lymph Nodes and Related Organs. Philadelphia, WB Saunders, 1985

Lawley TJ et al: A prospective clinical and immunologic analysis of patients with serum sickness. N Engl J Med 311 : 1407, 1984

Li FP et al: Malignant lymphoma after diphenylhydantoin (Dilantin) therapy. Cancer 36 : 1359, 1975

Masih AS et al: Rapid identification of cytomegalovirus in liver allograft biopsies by in-situ hybridization. Am J Surg Pathol 12 : 362, 1988

McFarland W and Schecter GP: The lymphocyte in immunological reactions in vitro: ultrastructural studies. Blood 35 : 683, 1970

Mroczek EC et al: Fatal infectious mononucleosis and virus-associated hemophagocytic syndrome. Arch Pathol Lab Med 111 : 530, 1987

Pattengale PK et al: Atypical lymphocytes in acute infectious mononucleosis. Identification by multiple T and B lymphocyte markers. N Engl J Med 291 : 1145, 1974

Royer HD and Reinherz EL: T lymphocytes: ontogeny, function, and relevance to clinical disorders. N Engl J Med 317: 1136, 1987

Salahuddin SZ et al: Isolation of a new virus, HBLV, in patients with lymphoproliferative disorders. Science 234 : 596, 1986

Saltzman RP et al: Disseminated cytomegalovirus infection—molecular analysis of virus and leukocyte interaction in virus. J Clin Invest 81 : 75, 1988

Severson GS et al: Dermatopathic lymphadenopathy associated with carbamazepine: a case mimicking a lymphoid malignancy. Am J Med 83 : 597, 1987

Stites DP and Leikola J: Infectious mononucleosis. Semin Hematol 8 : 243, 1971

Thorley-Lawson DA: Basic virological aspects of Epstein-Barr virus infection. Semin Hematol 25 : 247, 1988

VIII. Cellular Morphology of Body Fluids

Figure 54. Cerebrospinal Fluid. Artifacts and Curios. Reactive versus Malignant Lymphocytes.

Morphologic examination of cells in body fluids using Romanovsky panoptic stains has extended the diagnostic reach of hematopathologists into liquid recesses and sanctuaries once privy to cytology laboratories. Cerebrospinal fluid (CSF or spinal fluid) and fluid accumulations in the pleural, pericardial, and peritoneal cavities constitute tempting and accessible liquid biopsies, which are invaluable for tracking leukemias, staging lymphomas, and searching out carcinomatous dissemination. Air-dried Wright-Giemsa stained smears provide a level of definition and coloring unattainable with alcohol-fixed Papanicolaou (PAP) stained slides. The procedures are simple and performable in a single shift. Furthermore, "heme labs" are normally geared to apply adjunctive special staining methods needed for identifying cell lineages and useful in distinguishing neoplastic from reactive cells. Fortunately hematology and cytology laboratories are being drawn into ecumenism by shared dependence on contingent techniques, including electron microscopy, flow cytometry, and cytogenetics.

In CSF analysis, differential counts are performed on stained smears prepared from cell concentrates. Several methods are currently in use for concentrating cells from thin suspensions, the best of which are the *cytocentrifugation (cytospin) procedure* and the *Shen procedure*. When the white count is below 200 cells/µl and red counts do not exceed 5,000 cells/µl, cytocentrifugation is the procedure of choice, taking care to protect the cells by adding 2 drops of 22% albumin to 10 drops of well-mixed CSF in the cytocentrifuge cup. Gravitational force during cytospinning flattens and spreads cells, exposing and rearranging their parts. Nuclear segments of neutrophils are characteristically pushed to the periphery, an artifact that does not disguise their identity. Small lymphocytes, which comprise about two-thirds of cells normally found in the CSF, are spread out by the force of gravity so that the cytoplasm appears overly abundant, irregular, and eccentric. The loosened nuclei may reveal 1 or more of their submerged nucleoli, and mature lymphocytes at the outer edge of the cell button may resemble lymphoblasts (**Figure 54-1,** ×2,000). Monocytes, accounting for roughly one-third of cells in normal CSF, are severely but characteristically deformed in cytospin preparations: the cytoplasm is vacuolated and extends ragged or wispy processes, the nucleus is contorted into antic lobular shapes, and the pink granules are huddled in a paranuclear cluster at the cell center (**Figure 54-2,** ×2,000).

In patients who suffered cerebral or subarachnoid hemorrhage or endured a "bloody tap" between 4 days and several weeks earlier, the CSF may contain monocytes that were transformed into macrophages filled with *hemosiderin* (**Figure 54-3,** ×2,000). Hemosiderin granules stain dark blue or black in spinal fluid but have the same gravelly look as the green granules seen in iron-loaded macrophages of marrow (see **Figure 10-5**). Later, CSF hemosiderin is gradually converted to yellow or golden crystals of *hematoidin*, as shown in the spin-fragmented macrophage in **Figure 54-4** (×2,000).

The central canal system of the brain and spinal cord are lined by a monolayer of cuboidal epithelial cells known collectively as the *ependyma*. As ependymal cells lining the *choroid plexus* are exfoliated into the CSF, they cluster like cannonballs to form ominous purple aggregates that may alarm the unwary microscopist (**Figure 54-6,** ×2,000). Choroid plexus cells are most often seen in CSF obtained by cisternal or ventricular puncture. Like their paler cousins elsewhere in the ependyma, these cells are the size of large lymphocytes, but their nuclear chromatin is more smoothly homogeneous and nucleoli are absent. The exfoliated cells are tethered together by junctional complexes, and the outer aspects of cell clusters bristle with hairy villi.

Although blood or tumor cells obtained from spinal fluid and subjected to centrifugation may be flattened at their centers and scalloped at the margins, the outspread cells viewed against a water-clear background of dried spinal fluid often are more colorful and open to scrutiny than compatriot cells seen in blood smears. The color-coordinated mixture of reactive (transformed) and plasmacytoid lymphocytes in CSF from a child with viral meningitis (**Figure 54-5,** ×1,260) shows greater definition than the similar populations of blood cells portrayed in **Figures 52** and **53**. In leukemias, tumor cells may survive systemic chemotherapy, safe in their chemical concealment behind the blood : brain barrier. In acute lymphatic leukemia (ALL), lymphoblasts may first appear, or in relapse may first reappear, in CSF. Hence, therapy is tailored to "sterilize" leukemic enclaves that have claimed sanctuary in the central nervous system (CNS) and meninges. ALL lymphoblasts are seen in sharp and grim detail in the CSF of a young girl with CNS relapse in **Figure 54-7** (×2,000). In this cytospin preparation, every arch detail of malignant morphology is exposed, including abundant deep blue cytoplasm, bulky lobulated nuclei (with dysplastic indentations exaggerated by centrifugation), checkered chromatin, and prominent nucleoli coarsely framed in chromatin.

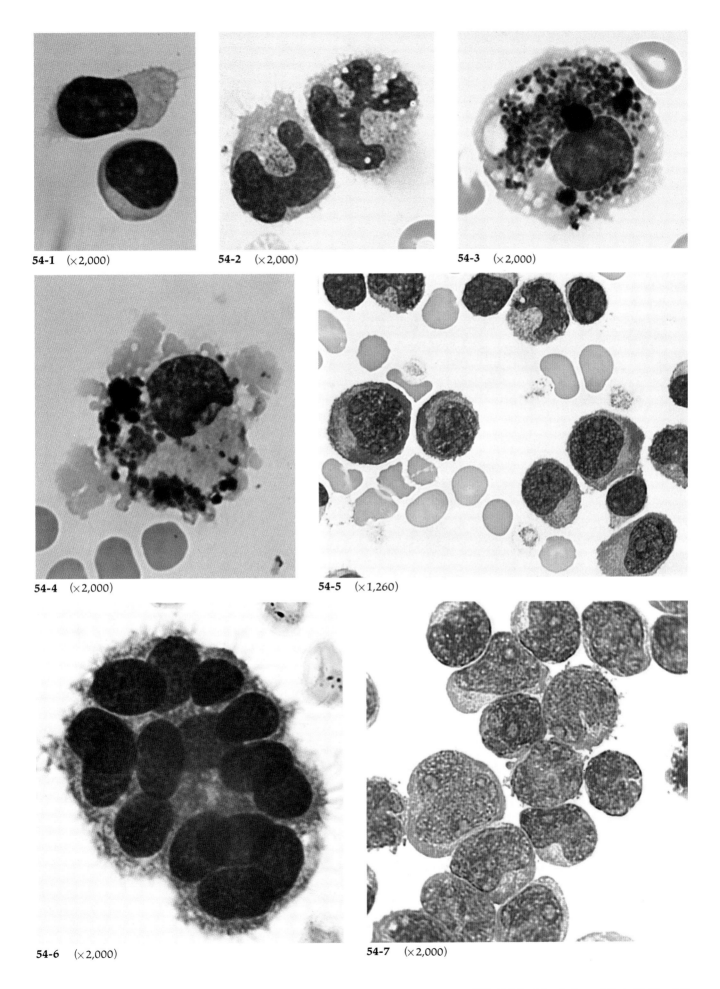

54-1 (×2,000)

54-2 (×2,000)

54-3 (×2,000)

54-4 (×2,000)

54-5 (×1,260)

54-6 (×2,000)

54-7 (×2,000)

Figure 55. Serous Fluid Morphology. Mesothelial Cells. Characteristics of Malignant Cells.

Serous effusions into pleural, pericardial, and peritoneal cavities can be rich in cytologic information, particularly if fluids are exudative and the urgent differential is between infection and malignancy. When white counts exceed 200/μl, this distinction leans heavily on the quality of smears made from cell concentrates. The most successful and simplest technique for obtaining undisturbed morphology is the *Shen procedure*, in which briefly spun cell buttons are tapped into suspension in 22% albumin, air-dried, and stained with Wright-Giemsa. The morphologist's first assignment is to recognize those innocent but intimidating creatures known as *mesothelial cells* (**Figure 55-1**, ×1,260). Mesothelial cells form the flat, epithelial pavement of visceral surfaces, but when desquamated into inflammatory fluids they fatten up and fuse into smoothly lobular aggregates. Ranging from 10 to 20 μm across, individual cells are spherical or egg-shaped, with gray–to–dark blue grainy cytoplasm that may contain multitudes of clear peripheral vacuoles. The nuclei are round or oblate and moderately variable in size, measuring half the diameter of the cell. Nuclear chromatin is dark purple and finely granular, and nucleoli are inconspicuous. Like their counterparts, the ependymal cells of CSF, mesothelial cells often sprout tiny projections and have a marked propensity to form cancerlike aggregates or to meld into molded syncytia, both social patterns being evident in **Figure 55-1**. Clusters or sheets of mesothelial cells and giant dark multinucleated agglomerates have an undeniably sinister look, but the uniform size and regular spacing of nuclei, absence of mitotic figures, and the "family similarity" between detached and coalesced forms distinguish them from clusters of malignant cells. When activated during inflammatory reactions, mesothelial cells enlarge, acquire plasmacytoid coloring, and project peripheral tags and microvilli, but nuclear structure remains bland and nucleoli are small and colorless (**Figure 55-2**, ×2,000). In **Figure 55-2**, the 2 large mesothelial cells at the top—one of them binucleate—immediately catch the eye, but it is the smaller immunoblast below, with its huge centroidal nucleolus, that threatens to take the patient's life. When tumor cells are in the minority, as in this pleural fluid from a patient with B immunoblastic sarcoma, immunophenotyping and cell-sorting technology are valuable aids. Mesothelial cells require close study because of their many guises and simulations. As mesothelial cells degenerate, their pyknotic nuclei drift off-center, creating imitations of plasma cells ("pseudoplasma cells"). Some decadent forms engage in erythrophagocytosis, mimicking macrophages, and all eventually fill up with a froth of vesicles as they expire.

In searching body fluid preparations for malignant cells, the first step is to hunt at low power for clusters, particularly for three-dimensional molded clumps (*ball formations*), and then to focus down to exclude mesothelial aggregates and examine for malignant features. The generic characteristics of malignant cells are largeness, pleomorphism, and a tendency to fuse. Nuclei are often very large and sometimes multiple, but variation in nuclear size is more telling than size alone. Tumor cell clusters often include pyknotic members, some of which are devoured by heartier neighbors in a fit of primitive cellular behavior known as *cannibalism*. Cannibalism and bizarre mitotic figures, 2 of the most deviant features of malignancy, are displayed in **Figure 55-3** (×800). Note the extreme variation in size among cells of this metastatic cluster, the overlapping disarray of the pleomorphic nuclei, several stages of cannibalism, and the three-way tie in metaphase. The cancerous features of anisocytosis, nuclear pleomorphism (*anisonucleosis*), and giant vacuolation are shown emphatically in the ascites fluid portrayed in **Figure 55-4** (×1,260). Note the unusual and irregular pseudopodal flaps at the margins of these breast cancer cells and the variable chromatin clumping and *hyperchromia* of the nucleus, a characteristic more visible in Papanicolaou-stained preparations. The renal papillary carcinoma cells in the pleural fluid shown in **Figure 55-5** (×1,260) reprise numerous markers of malignancy. The cluster of tumor cells at top are molded together, their outer margins are strangely darkened, and nuclear size, number, and deployment are in disorder. Several dark and shrunken cells in this unfriendly crowd appear to have been sentenced to programmed death, and the mesothelial bag at the bottom surrounds a banquet of cannibals feasting on their fallen cousins.

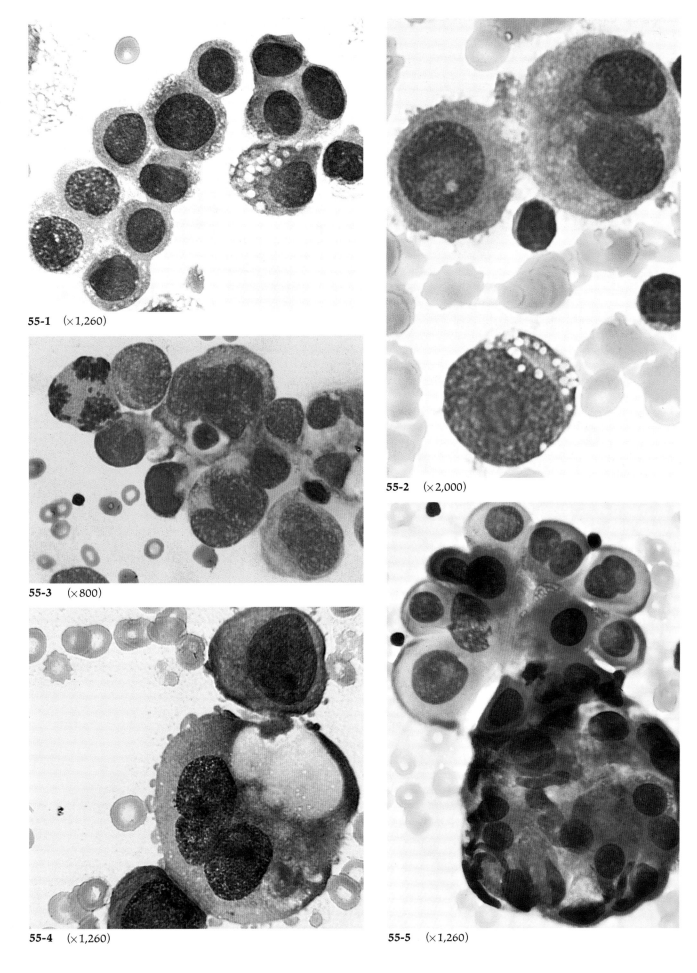

55-1　(×1,260)

55-2　(×2,000)

55-3　(×800)

55-4　(×1,260)

55-5　(×1,260)

Bibliography

Abrams J and Schumacher HR: Bone marrow in cerebrospinal fluid and possible confusion with malignancy. Arch Pathol Lab Med 110 : 366, 1986

Bia FJ and Barry M: Parasitic infections of the central nervous system. Neurol Clin 4 : 171, 1986

Bleyer WA et al: Reduction in central nervous system leukemia with a pharmacokinetically derived intrathecal methotrexate dosage regimen. J Clin Oncol 1 : 317, 1983

Boon ME et al: Qualitative distinctive differences between the vacuoles of mesothelioma cells and of cells from metastatic carcinoma exfoliated in pleural fluid. Acta Cytol 28 : 443, 1984

Carbone A and Volpe R: Cerebrospinal fluid involvement by malignant histiocytosis. Acta Cytol 24 : 172, 1980

Cheson BD: Clinical utility of body fluid analyses. Clin Lab Med 5 : 195, 1985

Choi HH and Anderson PJ: Diagnostic cytology of cerebrospinal fluid by the cytocentrifuge method. Am J Clin Pathol 72 : 931, 1979

Chou G and Schmidley JW: Lysis of erythrocytes and leukocytes in traumatic lumbar puncture. Arch Neurol 41 : 1084, 1984

De Ment SH et al: Diagnosis of central nervous system Toxoplasma gondii from the cerebrospinal fluid in a patient with acquired immunodeficiency syndrome. Diagn Cytopathol 3 : 148, 1987

Glass JP et al: Malignant cells in the cerebrospinal fluid (CSF): the meaning of a positive CSF cytology. Neurology 29 : 1369, 1979

Gondos B: Millipore filter vs. cytocentrifuge for evaluation of cerebrospinal fluid. Arch Pathol Lab Med 110 : 687, 1986

Goodson JD and Strauss GM: Diagnosis of lymphomatous leptomeningitis by cerebrospinal fluid lymphocyte cell surface markers. Am J Med 66 : 1057, 1979

Griffin JW et al: Lymphomatous leptomeningitis. Am J Med 51 : 200, 1971

Hoeltge GA et al: The differential cytology of cerebrospinal fluids prepared by cytocentrifugation. Cleve Clin Q 43 : 237, 1976

Homans AC et al: Immunophenotypic characteristics of cerebrospinal fluid cells in children with acute lymphoblastic leukemia at diagnosis. Blood 76 : 1807, 1990

Jay SJ: Pleural effusions, 2. Definitive evaluation of the exudate. Postgrad Med 80 : 181, 1986

Jellinger K et al: Primary intracranial malignant lymphomas: a fine structural cytochemical and CSF immunological study. Clin Neurol Neurosurg 81 : 173, 1979

Jellinger K: Primary lymphoma of the CNS. Arch Neurol 39 : 458, 1982

Kjeldsberg CR and Knight JA: Body Fluids, 2nd ed. Chicago, ASCP Press, 1986

Kolmel HW: Atlas of Cerebrospinal Fluid Cells, 2nd ed. New York, Springer-Verlag, 1977

Krieg AF and Kjeldsberg CR: Cerebrospinal fluid and other body fluids, in Clinical Diagnosis and Management by Laboratory Methods, 18th ed, Henry JB, Ed. Philadelphia, WB Saunders, 1991

Kruskall MS et al: Contamination of cerebrospinal fluid by vertebral bone-marrow cells during lumbar puncture. N Engl J Med 308 : 697, 1983

Kwee WS et al: Quantitative and qualitative differences between benign and malignant mesothelial cells in pleural fluid. Acta Cytol 26 : 401, 1982

Lauer S et al: Identification of leukemic cells in the cerebrospinal fluid from children with acute lymphoblastic leukemia: advances and dilemmas. Am J Pediatr Hematol Oncol 11 : 64, 1989

Lee HH et al: Early diagnosis of spontaneous bacterial peritonitis: values of ascitic fluid variables. Infection 15 : 232, 1987

Light RW et al: Cells in pleural fluid: their value in differential diagnosis. Arch Intern Med 132 : 854, 1973

Marsh WL Jr et al: Primary leptomeningeal presentation of T-cell lymphoma. Report of a patient and review of the literature. Cancer 51 : 1125, 1983

Pettersson T and Riska H: Diagnostic value of total and differential counts in pleural effusions. Acta Med Scand 210 : 129, 1981

Pui C-H et al: Central nervous system leukemia in children with acute nonlymphoblastic leukemia. Blood 66 : 1062, 1985

Raju RN and Kardinal CG: Pleural effusion in breast carcinoma: analysis of 122 cases. Cancer 48 : 2524, 1981

Sahn SA: Pleural fluid analysis: narrowing the differential diagnosis. Semin Respir Med 9 : 22, 1987

Saigo P et al: Identification of cryptococcus neoformans in cytologic preparations of cerebrospinal fluid. Am J Clin Pathol 67 : 141, 1977

Spriggs AI and Vashegan RI: Cytologic diagnosis of lymphoma in serous effusions. J Clin Pathol 34 : 1311, 1981

Stewart DJ et al: Natural history of central nervous system acute leukemia in adults. Cancer 47 : 184, 1981

Yam LT et al: Immunocytochemical diagnosis of lymphoma in serous effusions. Acta Cytol 29 : 833, 1985

A Glossary and Thesaurus of Hematologic Terms

Acanthocyte A spiny or spiculated red cell. The irregularly spaced spicules, lumps, and tassels connote an unbalanced surplus of membrane lipid, resulting in wrinkles and snags. Acanthocytes are prominent in spur-cell hemolytic anemia associated with severe hepatocellular disease and in abetalipoproteinemia. They appear in small numbers in all patients after splenectomy.

Alkylating agent An alkyl (hydrocarbon) free radical capable of substituting for a hydrogen atom is termed an *alkylating agent* when employed in therapy. The efficacy of alkylating agents in tumor therapy is due to their potential for causing covalent crosslinkage or other stable alterations in structures or enzymes essential to replication of DNA.

Alleles Two or more genes that occupy the same locus on homologous chromosomes. Autosomal chromosomes possess paired homologous genes. If the paired genes are identical, the individual is homozygous for the genetic character or protein product; if the paired allelic genes are not alike, the individual is heterozygous.

Allelic exclusion Normally at each immunoglobulin gene locus only 1 of the 2 allelic genes on homologous chromosomes is productive. This special exclusion prevents synthesis of hybrid antibody molecules having different specificities on each of the Fab halves. Monoclonal B cell populations disobey this exclusionary law, and either 1 or both alleles at the Ig locus affected may be rearranged.

Amyloid Double-stranded fibrillar protein formed by deposition of monoclonal free light chains (principally λ chains) which have undergone proteolytic degradation to fragments that collect in kidneys, liver, spleen, heart, and mesenchymal cells in general. Deposits of double-stranded AL fragments stain an amorphous pink with H&E, but under polarized light amyloid stained with Congo red dye emits a characteristic apple-green birefringence. Amyloidosis is a serious complication affecting about 10% of patients with myeloma.

Aneuploid, aneuploidy Cells having an abnormal number or variable number of chromosomes not a multiple of the haploid or diploid number. In describing a population of cells, the term is also applicable to partial aneuploidy, in which some cells have a normal complement of chromosomes and others have variable or abnormal numbers.

Anisocytosis Red cells of unequal size.

Asplenic states (asplenia) Absence of the spleen caused by surgery, atrophy, or congenital aplasia. Morphologic markers of asplenia include Howell-Jolly bodies, Pappenheimer bodies, acanthocytes, and giant platelets.

Auer rods Needle- or spindle-shaped cytoplasmic inclusions diagnostic of AML. Auer rods are stained red by Wright-Giemsa and can also be visualized by staining for myeloperoxidase, specific esterase, and PAS. Auer rods are fused cylindrical stacks of dysplastic primary granules and are particularly numerous in acute promyelocytic leukemia.

Azurophilic granule A cytoplasmic granule with affinity for methylene azure, becoming red or red-purple during Wright-Giemsa staining. The large (0.5 to 0.8 μm across), round or oblong, reddish granules of large lymphocytes, by convention, are termed *azurophilic*. When applied to the primary granules in immature granulocytes and monocytes, the expression *azurophilic* is confusing, and the term *primary granules* should be employed.

B cells Lymphocytes genetically programmed to produce antibodies. Immature B cells are formed in marrow, where they undergo Ig gene rearrangements and acquire surface IgM molecules that act as antigen receptors. Peripheral B cells exposed to their antigen of destiny transform to antibody-secreting plasma cells.

Band or band forms The preferred designation for young granulocytes, indicating an unsegmented neutrophil. Although entirely vernacular, the term *band* is less ambiguous and more descriptive than such unrecommended expressions as *stabs* and *juveniles*.

Barr body, Barr chromatin, or Barr sex chromatin body A small condensed mass of chromatin, representing an inactivated X chromosome, usually located just inside the nuclear membrane. Sex chromatin bodies are not found in normal males but appear in more than half of the somatic cells of normal females. The number of sex chromatin bodies per cell is 1 less than the number of X chromosomes. Among blood cells of normal females, Barr bodies are found primarily in neutrophils, approximately 2 or 3% of which display the characteristic drumstick appendage containing the condensed X chromosome.

Basophilic stippling Multiple small bluish freckles caused by clustering of blue-staining polyribosomes in immature red cells. Also known as *punctate basophilic stippling*. Basophilic stippling is seen in a small proportion of young red cells in many erythropoietic disorders, with the conspicuous exception of iron deficiency anemia. Pathologically coarse basophilic stippling is a characteristic but overpublicized feature of chronic lead poisoning, as only a minority of red cells (average, 2%, most of them reticulocytes) are heavily stippled. Lead inhibits the housekeeping enzyme, pyrimidine-5'-nucleotidase, which normally disposes of residual RNA at the time of nuclear extrusion. Coarse basophilic stippling also occurs in patients genetically deficient in this nucleotidase.

Bence Jones protein (BJ protein) Monoclonal free light chains found in the urine and serum of patients with myeloma. BJ proteins are detectable by heating or immunoelectrophoresis but do not register on the "dipstick" reaction used in routine urinalysis. Because of their small size, BJ proteins are readily filtered by renal glomeruli and are capable of causing severe nephropathy in patients with multiple myeloma.

Bernard-Soulier syndrome (BSS) A rare inborn disorder of primary hemostasis caused by a qualitative defect in platelets. BSS platelets lack a membrane glycoprotein (GPIb) that functions normally as a receptor for von Willebrand factor. Diagnosis is suggested by the large size of platelets and accounts for the alternative designation, *giant platelet syndrome*.

BFU-E (burst-forming unit—erythroid) Semicommitted stem cell capable of generating CFU-Es.

Blister cell Colloquialism for a red cell displaying clear outpouchings or "blisters." A membrane anomaly seen in certain hemoglobinopathies—especially sickle cell anemia and hemoglobin C disease—in which poorly soluble hemoglobin condenses beneath the cell surface.

Burr cell A round or ellipsoidal red cell having about a dozen smooth bumps spaced evenly around the margin. Unlike most echinocytes, these crenulated cells display central pallor. Burr cells are characteristic of uremia regardless of etiology, but their numbers do not correlate well with severity of either uremia or anemia.

Cabot ring A delicate violet or reddish ring form about 5 to 10 μm across, representing a vestige of the nuclear membrane persisting in young red cells. Shaped like hoops or figure eights, Cabot rings are seen only rarely, most often occurring in severe megaloblastic or hypochromic anemias.

cDNA Complementary DNA. DNA copied from an mRNA molecule.

CFU-E Committed stem cell capable of producing only erythroid cells, starting with proerythroblasts.

CFU-G Committed stem cell capable of producing solely myeloblasts. Parent to all granulocytes—neutrophils, eosinophils, and basophils.

CFU-GEMM Initialism for pluripotential myeloid stem cell. Forebear of granulocytes, erythroid cells, monocytes, and megakaryocytes.

CFU-GM Semicommitted stem cell capable of generating precursors of granulocytes or monocytes.

CFU-L Pluripotential ancestor of all lymphoid lines: B cells, T cells, and NK cells.

CFU-M Committed stem cell capable of generating only monocytes and their tissue forms, the macrophages.

CFU-Meg Committed precursor of megakaryocytes.

Charcot-Leyden crystals Needle-shaped bipyramidal bodies composed of crystalline lysophospholipase. These crystals are usually found in eosinophilic exudates or infiltrates of dysplastic eosinophils.

Chromatin The stainable components of a cell nucleus. On Wright-Giemsa staining, nuclear chromatin is violet, ranging in hue from lilac to purple. Chromatin is altered in its darkness or value by the quantity of basic histones included, the extent to which the fine strands of parachromatin are visible, and the extent of nucleoprotein condensation (nuclear pyknosis). The uncondensed, spread-out chromatin of immature cells is pale lilac; pyknotic nuclei are dark blue-purple or nearly black.

Chromosome banding Methodology for identifying chromosome segments involving use of selective stains. Giemsa ("G") bands appear when air-dried chromosomes are pretreated with trypsin. Fluorescent dyes such as quinacrine cause A-T base pair-rich striations to glow under ultraviolet optics. Other banding procedures include "R" banding (a complement to G banding) and silver staining for nucleolus organizer regions. Banding methods permit unequivocal identification of all chromosome arms and segments and enable tracking of abnormal chromosomal rearrangements.

Chromosome nomenclature Chromosome loci are indicated by specifying chromosome numbers, arms, regions, bands, and subbands. Chromosome number is identified by position in the idiogram: long arms are denoted by the letter q and short arms by p. Thus for region 3, band 2, of the long (q) arm of chromosome 14, the band is designated 14q32 (Burkitt's band), and the subband farthest from the centromere is denoted 14q32.3.

Chromosome rearrangements Numerical and structural gains, losses, and transpositions of chromosomes are denoted in shorthand by citing the kinds of aberration with a lowercase prefix, followed by the number, arm, and band of the chromosome affected. Gains or losses (deletions) are signified by plus or minus signs. Translocations are identified by the letter t, and the chromosomes and the arms and bands affected are paired within consecutive parentheses. The reciprocal translocation characteristic of Burkitt's lymphoma is designated as t(8;14)(q24.1;q32.3).

Clonal markers Monoclonal populations of cells can be identified by isozyme analysis (example: G6PD isozymes in heterozygous women), cell surface antigen markers, or monotonous TcR or Ig gene rearrangements. (See also **monoclonality**.)

Clone A colony or population of identical cells descended from a single ancestral stem cell. Normal cell populations are polyclonal with respect to their observable markers, their phenotypes. Phenotypic monoclonality suggests malignancy. Genotypic monoclonality (as in homogeneous expression of G6PD variants or of immunoglobulin rearrangements) is our best definition of cancer.

Cold agglutinins A solecism for *cold-active agglutinins*. Cold-active agglutinins are present normally in low concentration, reactive primarily with I or H antigens. In cold agglutinin disease, the titer of cold-active agglutinin—usually an IgM, κ chain type, with anti-I specificity—may be extremely high and cause cold-sensitivity reactions such as ischemic lesions in the acrocyanotic areas: the digits, ears, nose, and cheeks.

Colony-forming units Cell colonies derived in vitro from specified stem cells; each discrete colony is termed a *unit*. (See under **CFU**.)

Colony-stimulating factors

G-CSF Colony growth factor for neutrophils, released by monocytes and fibroblasts.

GM-CSF Colony growth factor for neutrophils, monocytes, eosinophils, and other myeloid cells, released by T cells, endothelial cells, fibroblasts, and macrophages.

M-CSF Colony growth factor for monocytes and macrophages, released by macrophages and endothelial cells. Also called **CSF-1**.

Coombs (antiglobulin) test Test for demonstrating attachment of antibodies or complement components to red cell surfaces. Heterologous (animal) antibodies to human immunoglobulins are used to bridge together cells coated with antibodies or other proteins too small to span cells directly. A positive *direct Coombs test* (direct antiglobulin test [DAT]) is essential to the diagnosis of immunohemolytic anemia. Agglutination can be hastened by light centrifugation ("spin Coombs test") or enhanced by combining PVP augmentation with use of an autoanalyzer. The *indirect Coombs test* detects antibodies floating free in plasma. Antibody in plasma in the absence of antibody bound to a patient's red cells is an *alloantibody*, not an autoantibody. The indirect Coombs test is of primary value in cross-matching before transfusion.

Crenated cell A categorical term for a red cell having numerous cornerlike projections; a cell puckered or desiccated so as to resemble a raisin.

Cytogenetics The art of chromosome analysis. Usually the chromosome constitution is ascertained by photographing a metaphase plate, cutting out the images, and arranging these in homologous pairs. This composite is known as the *karyotype*: the normal female diploid karyotype is denoted 46,XX, and that for males is 46,XY. Schematic representation of a karyotype in which images of chromosomes are arranged systematically according to length and centromeric position is an *idiogram*. (See also **chromosome banding**.)

Cytokines Hematopoietic hormones. Those that regulate myeloid and erythroid growth and differentiation are called *colony-stimulating factors.* Those concerned with immunity are named *lymphokines.* Lymphokines with established amino acid sequences are assigned interleukin (IL) numbers.

Cytoskeleton Articulated protein lattice of a cell that serves as a skeletal scaffold for the overlying lipid bilayer and integral membrane proteins.

Doubling time The time (Td) required for a mass of cells to double itself. Doubling time generally exceeds the potential doubling time predicted by the cell cycle time because of losses during cell division.

Drepanocyte A thin, elongated, fusiform, curved, falciform, sickle-shaped cell, often pointed or spiculated at 1 or both ends—usually alluded to simply as a *sickled cell.* The word *drepanocyte* is from the Greek *drepani,* meaning "sickle" or "scythe." Sickled-appearing cells, by whatever name, are diagnostic of sickle cell anemia or sickle cell variants.

Drumstick An ovoid sex chromatin body, about 1.0×1.5 μm across and attached by a slender stalk to an end lobe of the nucleus in a small percentage (usually 2 to 3%) of the neutrophils of normal females but not males. Drumsticks are equal in significance to Barr bodies. Apart from neutrophils, the only other blood cells that display sex chromatin bodies are eosinophils and possibly basophils.

Elliptocyte Red cell with an oblong, sausage, or canoe shape. The parallel sides and dumbbell distribution of hemoglobin distinguish elliptocytes from egg-shaped ovalocytes. A small percentage of normal cells are elliptical, but elliptocytes in excess of 10% indicate hereditary elliptocytosis.

Erythropoietin (EP or Epo) Colony growth factor for erythroblasts, synthesized by renal vascular endothelium. EP binds to receptors on CFU-Es, spurring these erythroid precursors to differentiate and divide. By radioimmunoassay, normal EP levels are 30 ± 7 mU/ml.

Exons Gene coding regions of DNA. Most coding regions are interrupted by noncoding DNA and by introns.

Fragmentation deformities Sufficient mechanical force splits red cells into 2 or more fragments or *schistocytes.* The usual products of cell cleavage, as occurs most spectacularly during microangiopathic hemolytic anemias, are a mixture of helmetlike or bib-shaped cells and small angular fragments. During intravascular coagulation, red cells draped over transverse fibrin strands slump 1 way or the other before cleaving along the axis of suspension. The unequal shapes created are half-spheroids (helmet forms) and kite-shaped fragments.

Gametocytes Sexual forms of malarial parasites, comprised of large distinctive macrogametocytes (females) and the smaller males (microgametocytes). Conspicuous but celibate while circulating in blood, gametocytes consummate their careers only if ingested by another mosquito, in whose covert cavern they mate and conspire to spawn infective sporozoites.

Genomic DNA All DNA sequences of an organism.

Golgi complex, Golgi apparatus An intracellular secretory organelle located adjacent to the cell nucleus, usually centroidally, occupying the hof, if one exists. Not visible by light microscopy, the Golgi complex is revealed by ultramicroscopy as consisting of complex saccules, vesicles, and canaliculi.

Graft-versus-host disease (GVHD) GVHD develops in all recipients of histoincompatible marrow and in about half of cases in which transplants are HLA-identical and mixed lymphocyte reaction-compatible. Acute GVHD occurs within 100 days and is dominated by confluent exanthem, watery diarrhea, and liver damage. Chronic GVHD emerges later as a multisystem collagen vascular disease.

Granules In hematologic argot, the term *granules,* unless otherwise qualified, alludes to the granular cytoplasmic inclusions that represent the logo of myeloid cells. During maturation, the first granules to emerge in abundance are coarse red-purple (azurophilic) bodies known as *primary granules.* Primary granules are synthesized only in promyelocytes and gradually diminish thereafter as the result of cell divisions and attrition. Primary granules contain myeloperoxidase and numerous hydrolytic enzymes. The smaller *secondary granules* (specific granules) appear in early myelocytes and are responsible for the faint lilac freckling of maturing neutrophils. Cytochemical staining for myeloid granules is the principal means for distinguishing myelogenous and lymphatic leukemias.

Gray platelet syndrome Rare congenital bleeding disorder caused by leaky platelets. Loss of α-granules during megakaryocyte maturation subverts aggregatory responses by platelets. These porous platelets are named for their bland (agranular) gray appearance on Wright-Giemsa stained smears.

Heinz bodies Rounded inclusions of precipitated hemoglobin visible by phase microscopy and made visible by supravital staining but not evident on Wright-Giemsa smears. Heinz bodies are an indication of oxidative injury as by exposure to oxidant drugs. Their presence insinuates the possibility of underlying susceptibility in the host in the form of G6PD deficiency or unstable hemoglobin disease. When Heinz bodies are expelled or forcibly torn from the red cell, diagnostic "bite-out" deformities are created.

HEMPAS An acronym for the type II variety of congenital dyserythropoietic anemia. The initials are derived from the diagnostic tongue-twister *hereditary erythroblastic multinuclearity (associated with a) positive acidified serum (test).*

Heterophil antibody A Forssman-type IgM antibody that agglutinates sheep or horse red cells and that appears during infectious mononucleosis (Greek *heteros,* "different, other"; and *philos,* "liking or having an affinity for"). Heterophil antibody can be distinguished crudely from other heterologous (interspecies) antibodies by differential absorption tests. Heterophil antibodies hemolyze beef (or ox) red cells and can be absorbed out by beef cells added in the absence of serum complement. Absorption with a paté of guinea pig kidney slightly diminishes heterophil levels of infectious mononucleosis sera but completely neutralizes the otherwise similar heterophil antibody that appears during serum sickness caused by injection of heterologous antitoxin. Agglutination of horse red cells by serum preabsorbed with guinea pig kidney is the most reliable and sensitive test for heterophil agglutinins. Unlike the persisting antibodies to Epstein-Barr virus that arise during infectious mononucleosis, heterophil antibody titers decline to low or undetectable levels within several months of infection.

Hodgkin's disease (HD): Ann Arbor staging classification

STAGE CHARACTERISTICS

I Involvement of a single lymph node region (I) or of a single extralymphatic organ or site (I_E).

II Involvement limited to 1 side of the diaphragm, either of 2 or more lymph node regions, or localized involvement of an extralymphatic site (II_E) plus 1 or more lymph node regions.

III Involvement of lymph node regions on both sides of the diaphragm, which may include localized involvement of an extralymphatic site (III_E) or spleen (III_S) or both (III_{SE}). (Stage III may be divided into: III_1, indicating that disease below the diaphragm is limited to the upper abdomen; and III_2, denoting para-aortic, mesenteric, iliac, or inguinal nodal involvement.)

IV   Diffuse or disseminated involvement of 1 or more extralymphatic organs or tissues, with or without associated lymph node involvement. The reason for classifying the patient as stage IV should be specified by identifying site with symbols. Hepatic (H) or marrow (M) involvement always indicates stage IV disease.

A   If asymptomatic.

B   If any of the following are present: unexplained loss of more than 10% of body weight in the preceding 6 months; unexplained fever, with temperatures above 38°C; night sweats; severe pruritus.

Howell-Jolly bodies   Dark purple, rounded inclusions, 1 to 2 μm across, representing fragments of pyknotic nuclear chromatin. Howell-Jolly bodies may appear in red cells during any process causing erythroid hyperproliferation. These chromatin inclusions are normally removed during splenic transit; hence, their unexplained presence is a marker of splenic absence or hypofunction.

Hyperdiploid   Applies to cells that possess more than the normal human complement of 46 chromosomes but, by inference, fewer than twice that number of any multiple thereof.

Hypersegmentation   Nuclear hypersegmentation, a term usually applied to neutrophils having an excessive number of nuclear segments or lobes. Neutrophils having 5 or more lobes are characteristic of megaloblastic anemia. Hypersegmentation may also affect other granulocytes and megakaryocytes and occurs as the result of 1 or more omitted terminal divisions.

Hypersplenism   A reduction in formed elements of the blood due primarily to increased splenic pooling. Better termed the *splenomegaly syndrome*, hypersplenism usually involves a moderate lowering of the levels of red cells, platelets, and, less regularly, white cells. Although cytopenia is seldom severe enough to warrant splenectomy, removal of the spleen in splenomegalic disorders almost always improves blood cell counts.

Hypochromia   Red cell pallor, indicative of a cellular deficit in hemoglobin.

Idiotype   The private antigenic profile of an antibody. The idiotype of an antibody is the aggregate of many individual antigenic determinants (idiotopes) in the variable region of the molecule. Being novel structures, antibodies themselves are immunogenic and stimulate corresponding immunoglobulins known as anti-idiotypes.

IL-1   Activates T cells, induces acute phase response, and mediates inflammation. Produced by macrophages.

IL-2   Autocrine growth factor for T cells expressing IL-2 receptors.

IL-3   (Multi-CSF) Supports growth of multipotent stem cells and acts in concert with CFU-GM to regulate pluripotential myeloid cells.

IL-4   Growth factor for activated B cells.

IL-5   Eosinophil differentiation factor.

IL-6   Acts in synergy with IL-3 and GM-CSF to amplify growth of myeloid cells.

IL-7   Stimulates growth and maturation of B cells and T cells.

IL-8   Stimulates neutrophil bactericidal functions.

Immunoglobulin gene rearrangements   Recombination events occurring early in B cell differentiation, during which variable (V) region genes are juxtaposed to diversity (D) and joining (J) genes, after which the VDJ complex is united with a constant (C) gene. Normally immunoglobulin (Ig) gene rearrangements are almost infinitely diverse. Amplification of a singular Ig gene rearrangement in a cell population is an indication of B cell malignancy.

Interdigitating cells   Specialized macrophages that function in the thymic cortex to remove and execute selectively young thymocytes and T cells that fail to display correct differentiation markers.

Interferon alpha (INFα)   Antiproliferative lymphokine, also known as *leukocyte interferon.* Recombinant INFα is useful in adjunctive therapy of certain chronic leukemias.

Interferon gamma (INFγ)   Antiproliferative lymphokine, also known as *immune interferon,* stimulates macrophage tumoricidal activity and prods B cells to transform into antibody-secreting plasma cells.

Interleukins   (See under **IL.**)

Introns   Noncoding intervening sequences (IVSs) of DNA that separate exons. Intron sequences must be cut out of mRNA transcripts to convert the transcript into an uncluttered exon continuum. Parts of excised introns possess RNA polymerase activity and are termed *ribozymes.*

Irreversibly sickled cells (ISCs)   Red cells that remain in a sickled shape despite oxygenation. (See **sickle forms.**)

Kappa/lambda analysis   Method for establishing clonality of B cell neoplasms by light chain analysis. Cells or M components that express or contain only kappa or lambda chains are monoclonal by definition. (See also **monoclonality.**)

Karyorrhexis   The process of breaking up or fragmenting the nucleus (Greek *karyon* + *rrhexis,* "a nucleus torn or disrupted"). Fragmentation, cleavage, or cloverleaf deformities of the condensed, pyknotic nucleus of mature orthochromatic erythroblasts are exemplary of the changes during karyorrhexis.

Karyotype   The chromosomal constitution or composition of a cell nucleus. Customarily, the karyotype is defined and displayed in a diagrammatic representation known as an *idiogram.* By convention, photomicrographs of metaphase chromosomes from a single cell nucleus are presented in a systematic array in which somatic chromosomal pairs are positioned in descending order of size and nearness to midposition of the centromere.

Keratocyte   A recently introduced term meant to describe red cells that possess pointed "horns." The term *keratocyte* (derived from the Greek *keration,* "a little horn"; or *keratos,* "the horned one, the devil") is used by some in reference to red cells bearing either 2 or more than 2 pointed processes ("horn cells").

Knizocyte   A hematologic neologism of uncertain etymology alluding to spheroidal red cells that are triconcave and bear a fleeting resemblance on scanning electron microscopy to a pinch bottle. On blood films, knizocytes look like the Greek letter theta). Knizocytes are minor anomalies sometimes seen in hereditary spherocytosis and immunohemolytic anemia.

Langerhans cells   A unique set of antigen-presenting cells that originate in marrow as monocytes, colonize the dermis, and travel to T cell zones of lymph node paracortex.

Langhans giant cells   Giant polykaryotic macrophages in which nuclei are arranged in a circular or horseshoe pattern surrounding a necrotic pool of offensive cytoplasm. Langhans-type giant cells are a conspicuous (but not singular) feature of mycobacterial infections. Langhans giant cells, which often contain 50 nuclei, are not to be confused with the mononuclear Langerhans cells of dermis.

Leukemogens Agents capable of causing leukemia. The best-documented leukemogens are ionizing radiations and alkylating agents used in chemotherapy. Both cause stable and unstable alterations and covalent crosslinkages in DNA that either kill or mutate marrow cells; the latter may lead to clonal proliferation.

Leukocyte alkaline phosphatase (LAP) More correctly termed *neutrophil alkaline phosphatase*. Neutrophil-specific enzyme of uncertain function, levels of which are characteristically low in chronic myelogenous leukemia (CML). Normally, more than 20% of mature neutrophils show strong LAP reactivity, but in 95% of CML patients enzyme activity is markedly diminished, LAP scores averaging about 13% of normal. Low LAP scores are characteristic but not diagnostic of CML, and scores may improve during intercurrent infections or pregnancy and following splenectomy.

Lymphokines Protein hormones that amplify or suppress growth, maturation, or activity of lymphocytes and certain other blood cells. Lymphokines are produced by lymphocytes, macrophages, endothelium, and other regulatory cells throughout the body. The term *lymphokine* encompasses interleukins, interferons, transforming growth factors, and tumor necrosis factors.

Lyonization X-linked genetic mosaicism in females resulting from random inactivation of the second (redundant) X chromosome of each diploid cell early in embryonic life. After lyonization, the female embryo becomes a mosaic of cells in which about half have an inactive maternal X chromosome (Xm) and the rest have an inactive paternal X chromosome (Xp). The inactivated X chromosome is visible as a heterochromatic pyknotic lump known in tissue cells as the *Barr body* and in neutrophils as the *drumstick*. Lyonization in which more or less than half of X chromosomes are inactivated is said to represent *extreme lyonization*.

M component Monoclonal protein manufactured by malignant plasma cells is often referred to as an *M component*. In multiple myeloma most M components are composed of a single heavy chain type plus a single light chain type. In 10% of myeloma patients the M component is entirely in the form of a monoclonal light chain, and, rarely, monoclonal proteins consist of isolated heavy chains (heavy chain disease). Some B cell tumors elaborate 2 or more monoclonal proteins arising from concurrent but independent clones.

Macro-ovalocyte Red cell that is both large and egg-shaped, the fused product of an omitted cell division. Macro-ovalocytes are pathognomonic of megaloblastic anemia. Also known as *oval macrocytes*. Ovalocytes should not be confused with elliptocytes.

Major histocompatibility complex (MHC) A supergene complex that codes from the polymorphic *HLA (human leukocyte-associated) antigens* found on all nucleated cells in the body. MHC genes are located on the short arm of chromosome 6, are inherited in codominant haploid packets, and are responsible for antigenic individuality. MHC and its HLA molecules identify self and nonself. Matchup between these "histocompatibility antigens" is necessary for organ transplantation.

Maurer's dots Relatively large, brick-red, irregular dots or spots often seen in red cells during falciparum malaria and occasionally seen in *Plasmodium malariae* infections. These dots are larger and less numerous than the Schüffner's dots of vivax malaria.

MCH Mean cellular (corpuscular) hemoglobin content. Computed by dividing the hemoglobin concentration of whole blood by the red cell count:

$$\text{MCH (pg)} = \frac{\text{hemoglobin (g/l)}}{\text{red cell count} \times 10^{12}/\text{l}}$$

The normal range is 28 to 32 pg.

MCHC Mean cellular (corpuscular) hemoglobin concentration, derived by dividing the hemoglobin concentration by the hematocrit value:

$$\text{MCHC (g/dl)} = \frac{\text{hemoglobin (g/dl)}}{\text{hematocrit (l/l)}}$$

The normal range is 32 to 36 g/dl.

MCV Mean cellular (corpuscular) volume, calculated by dividing the hematocrit by the red cell count:

$$\text{MCV (fl)} = \frac{\text{hematocrit (l/l)} \times 1,000}{\text{red cell count} \times 10^{12}/\text{l}}$$

The normal range is 83 to 99 fl.

M : E ratio (M/E ratio) The number of myeloid cells divided by the number of erythroid cells in marrow. M : E ratio is a crude index, informative only when cellularity of the specimen is good. Normally, the M : E ratio is about 3 : 1, but changes affecting both populations often blur interpretation.

Merozoite The small, mobile infective stage of protozoa, arising from schizogony.

Mesenchyma The primordial or embryonic cell population of the mesoderm, from which are derived the connective tissues, the blood vessels and hematopoietic cells, and the lymphatic vessels and lymphopoietic cells.

Mixed lymphocyte reaction (MLR) MLR (alias *mixed lymphocyte culture* [MLC]) is a sensitive typing test for compatibility at the HLA-D loci. Lymphocytes of the recipient are made unreactive by irradiation or mitomycin and then are coincubated with untreated responder cells from the donor. Donor T cells responding to HLA antigens of the recipient by enlargement, DNA synthesis, and division are predictive of graft-versus-host disease. An even more refined prediction pits cytotoxic T cells of the donor against the minor antigens of recipient's skin cells.

Monoclonality Monoclonality can be established by isozyme analysis or Southern blot analysis, the latter amplified, if necessary, by polymerase chain reaction technology. Restriction enzyme analysis by Southern blot technology registers the DNA profile of whole populations of cells and includes nonclonal with clonal contributions. More direct identification of a neoplastic clone of B cell origin can be achieved by immunofluorescent antibodies against an idiotypic determinant of surface immunoglobulin (sIg) molecules. Immunofluorescent staining for light chains is a widely used and important method in diagnosis of plasma cell disorders (see also **kappa/lambda analysis**).

Natural killer (NK) cells Heterogeneous subset of *large granular lymphocytes* (LGL cells). NK cells are recognized by their cargo of large azurophilic granules and by a surface glycoprotein, CD16. NK cells are capable of constitutive cytotoxicity.

Neutrophil alkaline phosphatase See *leukocyte alkaline phosphatase*.

Non-Hodgkin's lymphomas: histopathologic classification

CATEGORY	NEW FORMULATION	RAPPAPORT CLASSIFICATION
Low-grade	Small lymphocytic	Diffuse, well-differentiated lymphocytic (DWDL)
	Follicular, predominantly small cleaved cell	Nodular, poorly differentiated lymphocytic (NPDL)
	Follicular, mixed small cleaved and large cell	Nodular, mixed, lymphocytic and histiocytic (NM)
Intermediate-grade	Follicular, predominantly large cell	Nodular, histiocytic (NH)
	Diffuse, small cleaved cell	Diffuse, poorly differentiated lymphocytic (DPDL)
	Diffuse, mixed small and large cell	Diffuse, mixed, lymphocytic and histiocytic (DM)
	Diffuse, large cell: cleaved or noncleaved cell	Diffuse histiocytic (DH)
High-grade	Immunoblastic	Diffuse histiocytic (DH)
	Lymphoblastic: convoluted or nonconvoluted cell	Diffuse lymphoblastic (LB)
	Small noncleaved cell: Burkitt's or non-Burkitt's	Diffuse undifferentiated (DU)
Miscellaneous	Histiocytic	

Northern Blotting Method for identifying RNA fragments, analogous to Southern blotting of DNA. Useful in screening for major alterations in size and number of RNA transcripts.

Nuclear-cytoplasmic asynchrony, or dyssynchrony Imbalance between the growth and maturation of the nucleus and that of the cytoplasm. The expressions *nuclear-cytoplasmic asynchrony* (or *dyssynchrony*), *maturation arrest*, and *unbalanced growth* all allude to the same disordered process that is characteristic of megaloblastosis, in which nuclear and cytoplasmic maturation fail to proceed in tandem.

Nucleolus A rounded, clear, basophilic, RNA-rich organelle occurring singly or severally within the nuclei of immature cells during their early differentiation. Source of mRNA.

Oncogenes Highly conserved components (as proto-oncogenes) of the normal genome. Oncogenes participate in regulation of cell growth, but when displaced or damaged by translocation or mutation they are capable of inducing malignant transformation. Some oncogenes are under the control of recessively inherited regulatory genes dubbed *antioncogenes* or *tumor suppressor genes.*

Osteoclast activating factors (OAFs) Self-promoting cytokines secreted by lymphocytes and myeloma cells. The OAF tumor necrosis factor (TNF$_\beta$), alias *lymphotoxin,* is responsible for most of the bone destruction and hypercalcemia in multiple myeloma.

Pappenheimer bodies Red cell inclusions composed of aggregates of ribosomes, ferritin, and mitochondria. Pappenheimer bodies differ from basophilic stippling in being fewer in number and less evenly distributed; these inclusions are usually irregular, often form small clusters, and stain gray or blue-gray. Pappenheimer bodies are indicative of erythropoietic malfunction and are seen in megaloblastic anemias. Like Howell-Jolly bodies, they are also markers of splenic hypofunction or absence.

Platelet-derived growth factor (PDGF) A fibroblast mitogen found in megakaryocytes and platelets. PDGF is a transforming growth product of the C-*sis* oncogene located on the long arm of chromosome 22. PDGF is important in wound healing, but excessive leakage from dysplastic megakaryocytes, as in myeloproliferative disorders, causes myelofibrosis.

Poikilocytosis Descriptive of red cells having variable or irregular shapes.

Poly Laboratory argot for *neutrophil,* a nickname for *polymorphonuclear cell.* The term *neutrophil* is more explicit.

Polychromatophil A young anucleate red cell still possessing sufficient ribosomes to be faintly blue-tinged on Wright-Giemsa staining: that is, it displays polychromatophilia. The number of polychromatophils corresponds roughly to the number of reticulocytes.

Polychromatophilia A term usually applied to the cytoplasm of immature nucleated or anucleate red cells that contain both eosin-staining protein (hemoglobin) and ribosomes that stain with derivatives of methylene blue. The mixture of complementary colors gives the cytoplasm a grayed violet or muddy blue appearance. The expression *increased polychromatophilia* has a different connotation: it usually signifies an increased number of polychromatophils (see above).

Polymerase chain reaction (PCR) A powerful amplification method for enriching the yield of a known sequence of DNA, permitting analysis of DNA from small numbers of cells. After double-stranded DNA from a specimen is heated, the separated chains are allowed to bind to 2 oppositely oriented oligonucleotide primers that flank the ends of the targeted sequence. In the presence of a heat-stable DNA polymerase, the primers direct synthesis of new complementary strands, doubling the amount of target sequence. By use of automated thermal cyclers, this doubling process can be repeated 20 to 30 times within a few hours, yielding millionfold quantities sufficient for sequence analysis. PCR technology can be employed in identifying point mutations, clonal translocations, and clonal immunoglobulin and antigen receptor gene rearrangements. It is unrivaled in capacity for detecting sparse viral DNA sequences such as HTLV-I and in searching out and tracking clonal remnants following anticancer therapy. PCR technology is invaluable in performing rapid-readout prenatal diagnosis of genetic disorders.

Prolymphocyte Large, maturing, activated lymphocyte; an equivalent term is *immunoblast.* B prolymphocytes are immediate precursors of plasma cells and can be recognized by mature B cell phenotype (sIg⁺), darkly basophilic cytoplasm, and a single prominent medallionlike nucleolus. T prolymphocytes have scant cytoplasm, irregular nuclei, and T lineage markers.

Prussian blue stain A stain for nonheme ferric iron, as in ferritin and hemosiderin. In the prussian blue staining reaction, ferrocyanide reacts with ferric iron to yield the intense blue or blue-green pigment ferric ferrocyanide, $Fe_4(Fe(CN)_6)_3$. Prussian blue stain is particularly useful in staining the iron of siderocytes, ringed sideroblasts, storage and stromal iron, and iron in urinary sediments.

RDW Red cell size distribution width, a numerical expression quantifying anisocytosis, based on automated methods for assessing size variation in red cell populations. RDWs generate histograms (population profiles) that quantitate subpopulations of red cells having diameters below or above normal limits.

Restriction fragment length polymorphisms (RFLPs) RFLPs represent naturally occurring neutral variations in DNA fragment lengths that are inherited as codominant traits. Hence, Southern blot analysis of restriction enzyme digests of DNA can be used to establish gene linkage and inheritance. In parents who are heterozygous for a restriction site, RFLPs serve as classic mendelian markers. RFLP analysis for prenatal screening requires that the mother be heterozygous (informative) for the RFLP and that DNA be available from sufficient numbers of family members to assign linkage of 1 of the RFLP alleles to the suspect chromosome.

Retrovirus Virus particle composed of 2 identical subunits of single-stranded RNA genome imbedded in a core of protein and surrounded by an envelope of glycoproteins derived from the host cell. Once internalized by receptor-mediated endocytosis, genomic RNA is transcribed to DNA by means of its reverse transcriptase, and the double-stranded DNA product transcribes and multiplies RNA-containing virions that bud from the membrane and infect other cells. Human immunodeficiency virus (HIV) and human T cell lymphotropic virus (HTLV-I) are the most notorious retroviruses responsible for human disease. Both retroviruses are selectively infective for T4 lymphocytes. HIV uses the CD4 molecules on T4 surfaces as turnstiles for entering and devouring these essential lymphocytes.

Ring forms Early stage trophozoites formed by interiorized merozoites in malaria and babesiosis. Parasite DNA is in the red chromatin dot; the blue hoop-shaped ring is composed of RNA.

Ringed sideroblast (ring sideroblast) An orthochromatic erythroblast in which the nucleus is tightly surrounded by an arc or ring of coarse prussian blue–staining granules. A hallmark of sideroblastic anemias, ringed sideroblasts reflect a myelodysplastic derangement in heme biosynthesis.

Rouleaux Red cells stacked like dishes or coins (from the French for "packaged rolls of coins"). Rouleaux formation is induced by presence of linear or anisometric macromolecules and becomes striking at high concentrations of fibrinogen or immunoglobulins, particularly IgM. Unlike agglutinates, red cells clustered in rouleaux disperse when blood is diluted with saline. Rouleaux formation increases red cell sedimentation, and within limits the "sed rate" is an indirect measure of fibrinogen, immunoglobulins, and acute-phase reactants. (See **sedimentation rate**.)

Schizogony The process in the asexual stage of the malarial parasite whereby the daughter trophozoites, or schizonts, undergo segmentation into merozoites.

Schizont A sporozoan trophozoite that divides asexually by segmentation into numerous infective merozoites.

Schüffner's granules, or dots Fine, uniform, reddish granules or stipples observed in red cells infected with *Plasmodium vivax* or *P. ovale*.

Sedimentation rate Sedimentation rate (sed rate) or *erythrocyte sedimentation rate* (ESR) is an indirect measure of rouleaux formation and is used as an undependable (but strangely durable) test for inflammation. The principal causes of an elevated sed rate are increased levels of fibrinogen or of immunoglobulins (particularly IgM), but red cell settling is also profoundly affected by cell shape; hence, sed rates are accelerated by cell flattening and slowed down by spherocytosis. Sed rate is usually measured by the Westergren method, the simpler Wintrobe method, or the extravagant "zetafuge." The sed rate is a relic of galenism and should be replaced by direct measurements of parameters of inflammation, such as fibrinogen levels.

SEER Acronym for Surveillance, Epidemiology, and End Results Program of the National Cancer Institute. Rates and secular trends of cancer incidence and mortality are published annually by the American Cancer Society in the journal *CA*.

Shift to the left An unrecommended expression denoting a change or shift in the level of maturity of the cells specified. The intended meaning is that most cells in question show lesser maturity than normal and that there is a shift toward a younger stage. The expression *shift toward immaturity* is preferred.

Shift to the right Like the antithetical phrase *shift to the left*, this ambiguous expression, suggesting a shift toward an older cell stage, should be replaced by *shift toward maturity*.

Sickle forms Falciform elongation of red cells caused by extended polymerization of deoxyhemoglobin S. Patterns of deformation by polymer fiber growth depend on the rate and extent of O_2 unsaturation. Gradual polymerization generates well-aligned fibers to form classic "drepanocytic" sickle deformity. More rapid unsaturation creates a holly leaf pattern and, if deoxygenation is abrupt, a rigid "granular" discoid conformation is induced. In cells kept in a sickled position for long periods, membrane deformation is retained; the resultant *irreversibly sickled cells* (ISCs) account for most sickled forms seen on air-dried blood smears.

Siderocytes Red cells containing iron-staining (siderotic) granules. Unlike Pappenheimer bodies, siderotic granules are visible only if stained specifically for iron with the prussian blue reaction. Siderocytes are found in many hematopoietic disorders, particularly sideroblastic anemias, but are much less prevalent than Pappenheimer bodies. Siderocytes appear in abundance only after splenectomy.

Southern blotting Technology for identifying DNA fragments following cleavage by 1 or more restriction enzymes. Separated fragments hybridized to a specific DNA probe can be used to locate and characterize specific genes.

Spherocyte A spherical or spheroidal red cell, a morphologic hallmark of hemolysis. Spherocytes lack central areas of pallor and are increased in thickness and diminished in diameter: hence they appear small and dark. Spherocytosis occurs when surface membrane area is decreased relative to cell volume. Accordingly, spherocytes reach their limiting (hemolytic) volume when suspended in saline that is only slightly "hypotonic" (hypo-osmolar) and therefore are described as showing increased *osmotic fragility*. Spherocytosis is most uniformly evident in hereditary spherocytosis and immunohemolytic anemias, but nearly all hemolytic disorders are associated with some spherocytes.

Splenic red pulp Highly vascular intermediate and distal portions of splenic microvasculature, composed of 2 alternating structures: *splenic sinus* es and *splenic cords*. Red pulp is the filter of the bloodstream.

Splenic white pulp Resting place for T cells and secondary source of B cells. White pulp includes transient aggregates of recirculating T cells that are skimmed from circulation to form the periarterial lymphatic sheath, and spherical foci of B cells, which form primary and secondary follicles. T cells rest up in the spleen; B cells proliferate there.

Sporozoite The small forms of *Plasmodia*, liberated from the oocytes in the anopheles mosquito and concentrated thereafter in that pest's salivary glands. Sporozoites are introduced into the human bloodstream when the female mosquito takes in a blood meal. Thereafter, they mature in the liver to become trophozoites infective for red cells, and these in turn either change into mature schizonts that fragment into merozoites or become gametocytes. The former massively spread infection to other red cells; the latter, if ingested by another female mosquito, complete the parasitic cycle by mating in the blood-filled abdomen of the mosquito and producing a new batch of infective sporozoites.

Stab (stab form) Laboratory patois for *band form neutrophil*. Neither descriptive nor recommended.

Stem cell factor (SCF) Growth factor for multipotential stem cells, secreted by marrow stromal cells.

Stem cells A class of cells having 2 generative capabilities: replication and formation of more-differentiated offspring.

Totipotential stem cell A cell capable of generating any of all cell lines of which the species is genetically capable. The only true stem cell is formed by the fusion of 2 gametes at conception. The term *totipotential* overstates the capabilities of hematopoietic stem cells.

Multipotential stem cell The highest echelon stem cell of marrow, capable of spawning pluripotential precursors of all myeloid and lymphoid lineages.

Pluripotential stem cell A midechelon stem cell, ancestor of committed myeloid and lymphoid cell lines.

Unipotential stem cell Precursor committed to differentiate into a single hematopoietic cell line.

Stomatocyte A red cell, usually somewhat spheroidal, that in suspension resembles a bowl or folded cup and on a smear possesses a slotlike area of central pallor. The resultant pattern is often reminiscent of a mouth: thus the term *stomatocytes*, from the Greek *stomata* ("mouths") plus *kytoi* ("cells"). Stomatocytes may be the predominant cells in hereditary stomatocytosis, a syndrome comprising a group of rare, usually hemolytic, membrane disorders.

Stroma Matrix of adherent multilayered cellular complex that provides the microenvironment for hematopoiesis. Composed of endothelium, fibroblasts, reticular cells, fat cells, and macrophages. Furnishes lodging and issues short-range growth factors.

Supravital Denoting staining of intact and unfixed cells, usually while in free suspension after their removal from the bloodstream or from body fluids.

Target cell A red cell in which some or most of the hemoglobin centralizes as the cell is air-dried on a coverslip or slide, thereby conferring a targetlike or bull's-eye pattern. Targeting is a drying artifact that occurs in cells that are abnormally broad or in which the hemoglobin (e.g., hemoglobin C) is poorly soluble. During drying, targets are puddles of hemoglobin left behind in the molecular rush toward the fullness of the red cell rim.

T cell receptor rearrangements DNA coding for T cell antigen receptors (T cell receptors or TcRs) is rearranged from V, J, and C region gene segments in a manner analogous to Ig gene rearrangements. Singular TcR gene rearrangements uniformly shared in cell populations are characteristic of T cell malignancies.

T cells Lymphocytes genetically programmed to become equipped with T cell antigen receptors (TcRs). Mature T cells employ their TcRs to recognize antigen that is presented by macrophages or B cells: hence T cells are responsible for cell-mediated (cellular) immunity. All T cell functions involve reactions on the surfaces of cells.

Teardrop form Red cell with a tapered or droplike shape. Classicized by some as a *dacryocyte*. Teardrop shape is acquired when red cells are subjected to prolonged tugging, as when cells loaded with inclusions attempt to slither through the splenic cords. Teardrop forms are most numerous in thalassemia or myelofibrosis but disappear after splenectomy.

Thesaurocyte An imaginative expression depicting any and all of the various kinds of storage cells seen in the marrow in lipid storage diseases, mucopolysaccharidoses, chronic myelogenous leukemia, and many other disorders in which macrophages become stuffed with undigestible macrometabolites (Greek *thesaurus* plus *kytos*, "treasure cell").

Torocyte A ring-shaped red cell in which all of the hemoglobin is distributed in a narrow peripheral rim, leaving a large colorless central area. The term *torocyte* (Greek, *toros*, "to pierce") is employed by some as a synonym both for flat, pale-looking cells (leptocytes) and for target cells. Torocytes may be seen in hypochromic anemias, particularly thalassemia. The term is best reserved for reference to the stark, ring-shaped red cells seen as a desiccation artifact.

Trophozoite Asexual ameboid form of malarial plasmodia occurring during erythrocytic phase of malaria. Trophozoites are derived from intracellular ring-stage forms and multiply through schizogony.

Variant lymphocyte A term recommended mainly as an alternative to the indiscriminate expression *atypical lymphocyte*, which traditionally has encompassed normal large granular lymphocytes (NK cells) and prolymphocytes. Variant lymphocytes comprise all forms of nonnormal lymphocytes, including those seen in drug reactions and viral infections. If either term (*variant* or *atypical*) is used, the morphologic specifics of the aberration should be stated.

Index

Index